WHAT'S IN YOUR SHOES?

101 Solutions for Foot Pain on a Budget !

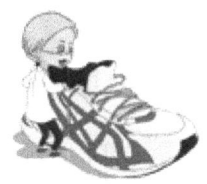 

I0426581

By **Lynda Elliott Goyzueta**

www.FootFixes.com

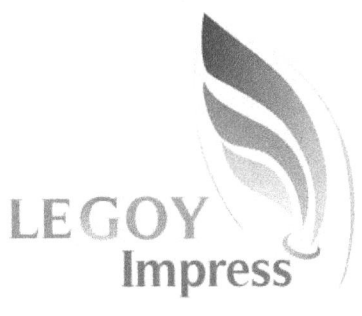

Important Disclosure

All rights reserved

ISBN-13: 978-1492311423 (pbk)
ISBN-10: 1492311421 (pbk)

Credits

Danielle Steinfeld............................Editor
Mr. Kenny Abigael U. Badana ....Illustrations
Vikiana Bulgaria..............................Cover Design
JD Moore of Moorefficient..............IT Support
Roque Goyzueta..............................Format

Printed and Bound by Legoy Impress
Manufactured in the United States of America

First Edition

I dedicate this book to my:

...children and their spouses, Sherry & Dewey, JD & Asia, and Angela & Bill, my warriors of support.

...Mother and Dad; I still miss our phone calls and know you are proud of me.

...Aunt Madge, who is a great example of positive attitude.

...editor, Danielle Steinfeld. You are amazing! I am lucky to have you as a friend as well.

Most of all, to my husband, Roque Goyzueta, who always believes in me; I am a lucky woman indeed. Thank you for all the time you spent with me at Starbucks (my best place to write).

CONTENTS

INTRODUCTION

When I met Lynda, she was working in an orthopedic shoe store. What I saw from the beginning was her special kindness and care with the clients. Her professionalism and sweet way to handle the patient's problems earned her the nick name of 'My Angel', as well as receiving many compliments cards and recommendations.

This book is the final result of months of hard work, researching her archives and planning an easy way to reach the people without losing her narrative style but being useful to helping people with foot problems.

In the first part, called "What's In Your Shoes", Lynda describes several real stories and gets the reader involved and, in many cases, identifying with the patient. This part helps the reader understand the collateral issues that people with foot problems have and how, many times, they prefer to hide it.

The second section of the book is called "101 Solutions for Foot pain on a Budget" and it is in this part where Lynda gives practical and inexpensive ways to alleviate foot problems.

In summary "What's in your shoes" is a good guide to understanding and helping people with foot problems; made in an easy language with entertaining and didactic stories.

Roque Goyzueta
International Security Consultant
Husband and happy patient

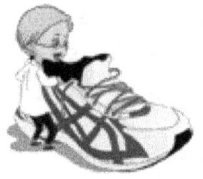

WHAT'S IN YOUR SHOES?

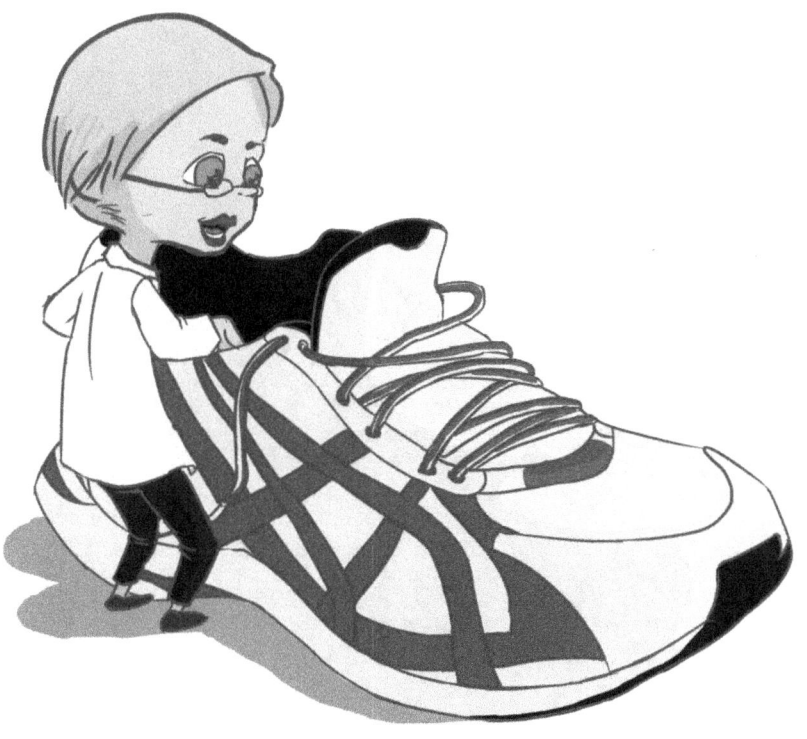

Meet Little Lynda

These characters are based on the author, Lynda Elliott Goyzueta, Certified Pedorthist.

Each "Little Lynda" has a purpose and personality.

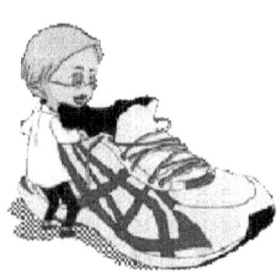

What's in your shoe?

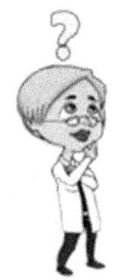

"I'll have to think about that"

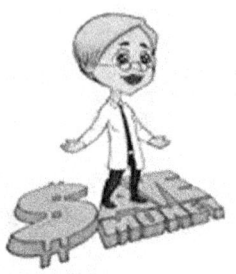

"SaveMoney"

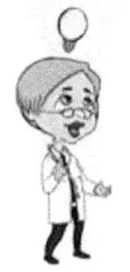

"Eureka! I have an Idea!"

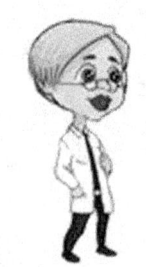

"This is serious"

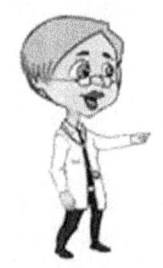

"Note important point"

Chapter 1

Pedor What?

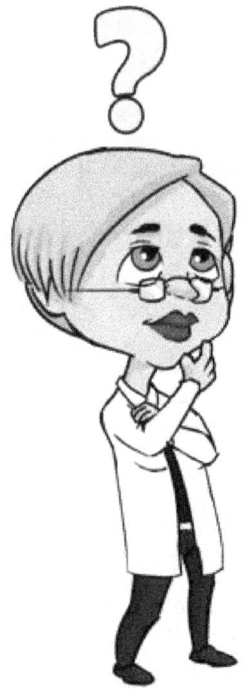

"My feet are still on the ground. I'm just wearing better shoes."

—

Oprah Winfrey

Have you ever found a surprise, like a Kotex pad, in someone's shoe? How about a piece of a cardboard beer box cut into a horseshoe shape? What people hide in their shoes is incredible.

Urban legend claims that Marilyn Monroe had six toes. Many would argue that anything looked good on Marilyn!

Is your second or third toe longer than your big toe? Really push those toes flat to compare. The longer second toe is called a "Morton's" toe. It is supposed to be a sign of leadership and strength. Your destiny can be tied to just the right pair of shoes. Just ask Cinderella!

People are always trying new things to get comfortable. Many serious foot problems cannot be solved without medical intervention. We can do many things ourselves with common materials and a little inventive creativity.

When was the last time you fixed or invented something yourself?

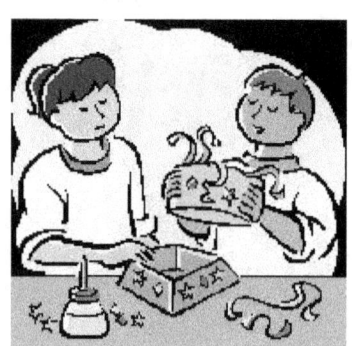

Was there a time when you did not:

- Throw it away
- Call a handyman
- Ask your significant other to fix it

- Or take it to the repair service?

With a little imagination, asking questions, reading books, and watching YouTube, it is amazing what we can do. Trial and error are best buddies!

Surprise yourself and those around you who think you have lost your creative spirit! You may save some money too!

Custom-made orthotics can be very expensive, especially if you are living on a fixed income, such as unemployment insurance, SSDI, or Social Security benefits. Many people can't afford them no matter how badly their feet, legs, ankles, knees, hips, back, neck or jaw hurts. So, what do they do? They find ordinary things to ease their discomfort.

I am an ABC Certified Pedorthist.

"What in the world is that?"

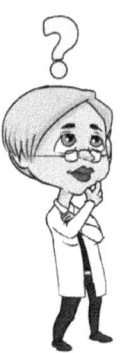

*"A **Certified Pedorthist** is a health care professional who manages comprehensive pedorthic patient care. This includes patient assessment, formulation of a treatment plan, implementation of the treatment plan, follow-up and practice management ...*

Certified Pedorthists work with patients and their footwear to conform to a doctor's footwear prescription as part of the patient's treatment."

—*The **A**merican **B**oard for **C**ertification in Orthotics, Prosthetics & Pedorthics*

"Whew! Pedorthic devices; what does that mean?" If it can prevent or alleviate a foot problem, it could even mean a *Kotex pad!*

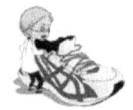

Orthopedic: *"Given the original Greek roots, the term means "to straighten the child" and refers to the orthopedist's specialization in correcting crooked or broken bones."*

—Dawn Walls-Thumma, editor for **Bartleby** and **Antithesis Common**

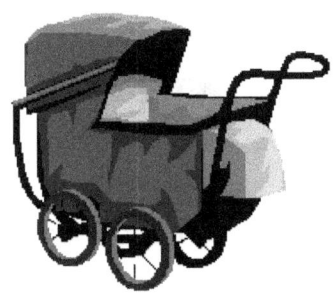

Baby Pedorthist

I began my career unofficially in 1952, when I was a baby. My mother's breast milk did not have enough nutrients to feed a growing baby. Following all of the old wives' tales, she drank beer, ate Tums, and took vitamins to increase the quality and nutrition of her breast milk.

"You would hang your bottom out the window if it would help your breast milk." My pediatrician, Dr. Donovan laughed. He knew Mother was desperate.

I developed *Rickets*.

"Rickets is the softening and weakening of bones in children, usually because of an extreme and prolonged vitamin D deficiency."

—Mayo Clinic

My bones were bendable like a soft chicken's wishbone. Walking at nine months of age; my skinny legs were as bow-legged as a cowboy riding a big fat horse.

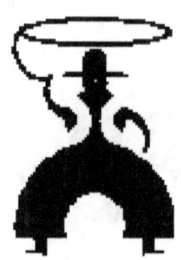

Bow-legged Cowboy

Dr. Donovan prescribed a diet of liverwurst balls and Dr. Pepper. Liverwurst was full of iron and vitamin D. Dr. Pepper was made from real prune juice back in the 1950s. My bones became strong and straighter.

As I grew, I walked splayfoot, like a duck, with toes pointed out and arches flat. This took a toll on the development of my knee joints.

On my tenth birthday, I was presented with ten-pound (*slight exaggeration*) saddle oxfords. They were black and white leather with fat shoe strings and a steel shank under the arches; I wore them every day of my life for two years.

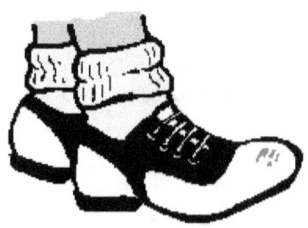

Orthotic Saddle Oxfords

The orthopedic shoe clerk showed me how to put a "cookie" in my shoe—a compressed cotton, half-moon pad worn under my arches. With an adhesive, the cookie was attached to the shoe under the shoe liner.

My knees would ache each night as my legs were adjusting to the new way to walk. My mother would massage my legs and drape them with hot towels so I could sleep. "Thanks Mother!"

My legs became straight. Strangers in airports would watch and tell me how gracefully I walked. This improvement was brought about slowly with the aid of **foundational support and structured devices**. It was my first experience using an **orthotic device.**

Little did I know I would have a career one day using devices similar to those heavy black and white shoes!

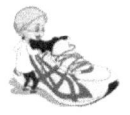

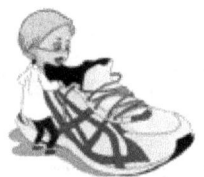

Chapter 2

Is This Shoe Right for You?

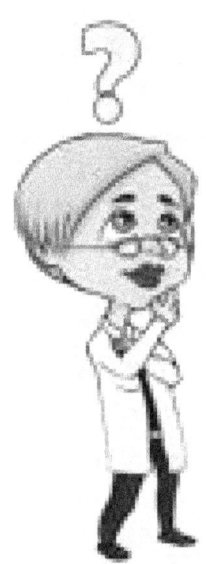

"One in two women own more than 30 pairs of shoes."
—
Harper's Bazaar

What shoe makes you think of an African tribe?

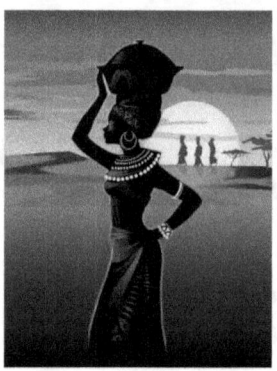

Central African Tribe

I sold the famous **Rocker Bottom** line of shoes at a retail shoe store. These were special shoes that need demonstration and education. Anyone selling them was taught to practice with customers so that they could walk in them.

The normal way to walk with a heel landing and toe push-off in a flat bottom shoe does not apply with these shoes.

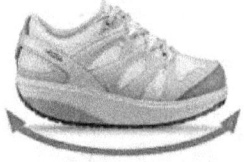

Rocker Bottom Shoe

I sold hundreds of these $200-$300 shoes. The original design came from a European creator, but was based on the posture, lack of foot and back problems, and high mobility of a tribe in central Africa.

This tribe has a reputation for walking long distances without rest or fatigue. They typically walk barefoot on soft, springy surfaces. The idea was that the instability of walking on surfaces like sand, peat-moss or soft earth contributes to better posture and improves muscle strength.

There is still a controversy over the benefits and liabilities of this shoe design. One of the real problems I saw working in a retail shoe store was the push to make a sale based on *"medical-sounding advice."*

Much of the literature and training was focused on balance, as in, "wearing these shoes will improve your balance." What section of the population do you think of most when you think of 'poor balance'?" Our balance can deteriorate as we age due to illness, injury, or simple lack of exercise.

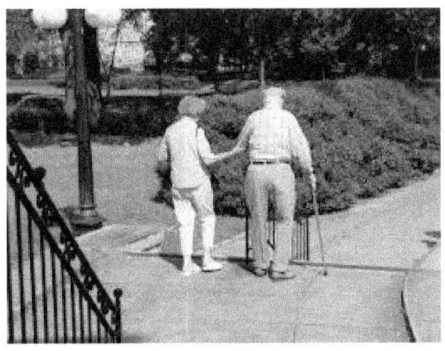

Elderly with poor balance

An elderly woman, walking with a cane, came to the shoe store on my day off. She was 76 years old with very poor balance. After reading an article in a magazine that said, "Rocker Bottom shoes can improve your balance," she wanted a pair.

Unable to walk without her cane, this elderly woman depended on two employees working at the shoe store for support. As she stood up in the Rocker Bottom Shoes, the employees held each of her hands as she tried to walk about 15 feet from a chair to the counter.

The employees spent about thirty minutes walking around with her until she paid for the shoes and left. The male clerk carried them to the car for her. These employees rang up the shoes and got credit for the sale. The Rocker Bottom shoes cost about $300.

The elderly woman's daughter came to the shoe store about six months later. You could see the frustration on her face.

"Mother worked hard with those Rocker Bottom shoes to get her balance, but gave up after a few days. Mother's shoes sat in the closet until the day she went to live in the nursing home." I couldn't believe she spent so much on them. She couldn't walk without her cane and it seems the people selling the shoes to her could see that. "Her doctor was very upset with her." The daughter explained.

Unfortunately, the daughter had waited too long, and with the store owner's policy, there was no chance to get her mother's money back.

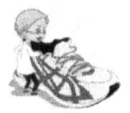

On the other hand, a well-known **Denver metals artist** regularly bought the Rocker Bottom shoes for himself and his assistants. Working in a foundry, he firmly believed in the support and cushion of the shoes.

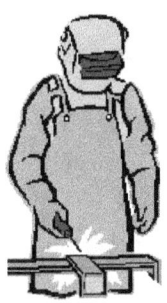

Metal welding artist

Standing on concrete day after day put a lot of pressure on the artist's feet and back. In this situation, the shoes' cushioned bottoms were an excellent choice.

Every six months the artist would come in and buy another six pairs of shoes. He was a very talented artist, so money was not an issue, and he was happy to buy them for his employees.

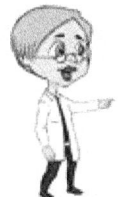

Not every solution is right for every person. It can depend on how much disposable income you have and how well you deal with change. Your medical needs can be determined by your health care professional.

Rocker Bottom shoes are often used in orthopedic settings, but the position of the rocker, height, depth, and materials vary according to needs.

If someone has a broken toe, frequently a physician will order a healing shoe or boot that has a rocker bottom to keep the toe straight and rigid in a cast.

The same is true for ulcers caused by diabetic side effects; the pressure must be off-loaded for healing to take place.

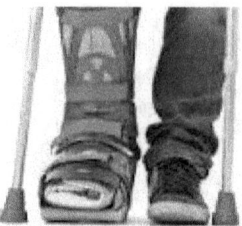

Rocker Bottom walking boot

A warning should be put on the outside of the shoe box: *Do not wear these shoes on a ladder or while roofing a house.* Yes, I had customers who attempted to do this and had to be treated for injuries.

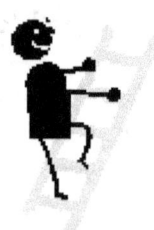

Climbing a ladder wearing Rocker Bottom shoes

The following examples are of real people and real events

Bunny Baker (her stage name) was beautiful, blonde, and vivacious. She was visiting from Las Vegas, Nevada. Bunny had been invited to a celebrity wedding and wanted to wear what she called her Las Vegas "stripper" heels. The shoes were completely clear, with high heels and no back straps.

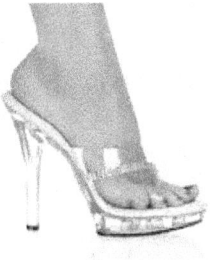

Open back high heels

She was so excited and animated that I didn't notice her problem until she tried on her shoes. One foot was three sizes smaller than the other!

If I filled up the end of the shoe to keep her smaller foot from sliding forward, the padding would show through the clear shoes. If I let the foot slide forward and tried to tighten the front of the shoe, the arch would be in the wrong place and would cause her pain.

We were both feeling frustrated as I really wanted to help this woman; but there was nothing I could do but suggest she try another store.

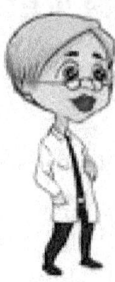

Bunny's problem with "stripper heels" might be superficial by our vanity standards, but to her, this problem robbed her of feeling "normal." Self-esteem is an important part of who we are and how we feel.

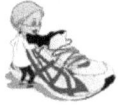

Some foot and shoe challenges involve employment. **Denver International Airport** has jobs that require solid black shoes, such as flight attendant. Flight attendants often came to my store with tales of woe about their legs, feet, knees, back, and shoulders.

They firmly believed that the marble/granite floors were harder, with less flexion than concrete. The attendants really wanted a more cushioned, supportive shoe, so they would choose a more athletic or walking shoe style. We had no problem finding good shoes that were solid black leather that would work with their uniforms, but the shoes had to be *solid* black. All the shoes we could find had some identification tags, emblems, or logo designs with text and color.

The flight attendants were very disappointed until I brought out a permanent black magic marker and colored in the designs. Now they were solid black and would meet the dress code. Problem solved!

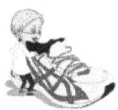

Mr. Granby was a well-respected attorney for many years. As a trial lawyer, he spent several hours each day on his feet fighting for his clients, speaking before a judge and jury.

His clothing needed to show the public that he was a serious man. Mr. Granby projected wisdom and education; therefore, professional attire was always a requirement (as well as his preferred way) in presenting himself.

I liked him right away. He had a generous smile, sandy-blonde hair, and a warm laugh. It was hard to picture him as a stern and aggressive trial lawyer.

While I sat on my 'fifteen-inch shoe-fitting stool', Mr. Granby told me about his pain and the problems he was having getting comfortable shoes. I took off his shoes and socks and saw that his right foot was flat; it was more than low arches; much more.

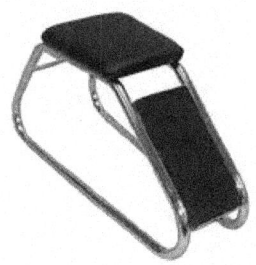

Fifteen-inch shoe-fitting stool

I had never encountered his condition before. Most of our customers had a more common problem, like sore arches, painful heels, or a wish to find a better athletic or walking shoe. This was different than helping him pick out a comfortable pair of shoes to fit his lifestyle.

At that time I didn't know the name or cause of his condition (PTTD or *Posterior tibial tendon dysfunction*).

Posterior tibial tendon dysfunction *is one of the most common problems of the foot and ankle. It occurs when the posterior tibial tendon becomes inflamed or torn. As a result, the tendon may not be able to provide stability and support for the arch of the foot, resulting in flatfoot....*

An acute injury, such as from a fall, can tear the posterior tibial tendon or cause it to become inflamed. The tendon can also tear due to overuse. For example, people who do high-impact sports, such as basketball, tennis, or soccer, may have tears of the tendon from repetitive use. Once the tendon becomes inflamed or torn, if not treated, the arch will slowly fall (collapse) over time.

—OrthoInfo (Member of <u>AAOS American Academy of Orthopedic Surgeons</u>)

Mr. Granby's ankle had bent inward and his arch appeared to be like another heel sticking widely out of his foot.

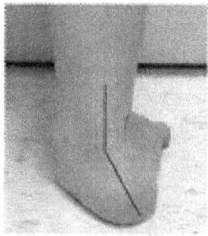

Flat arch, valgus heel (PTTD dysfunction)
(This picture is taken from the back of the heel. The black line was drawn to show the angle of the ankle and foot)

I was choking back the "How the heck am I going to help this man?" I had no shoes in the store shaped like his foot, nor any that were wide enough. Even if they were wide enough, the arch and shape of the shoes would be all wrong for his ill-formed feet.

Just trying a normal shoe on his foot put too much pressure on his collapsed arch bones. There was only skin between his arch bones and the floor. Then there were his toes. They all curved dramatically toward the outer side of his foot and he couldn't push forward properly on his big toe.

When a patient has posterior tibial tendon dysfunction (PTTD) with a flatfoot deformity, the front of his foot points outward. The 'too many toes' medical sign happens when even the big toe can be seen from the back of the patient's foot.

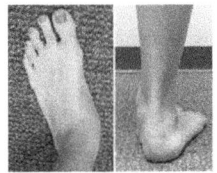

"Too many toes" medical sign

(The picture on the right is taken from the back of the heel)

I showed him step by step where I saw the problems with fitting him. Even in a protective pair of shoes I was afraid that he would develop blisters and worse, possibly ulcers.

He was well aware of his condition and very patient. Mr. Granby encouraged me to keep trying as he had tried everything he could to get help from other professional shoe fitters.

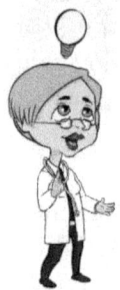

An idea struck me that might just work! I could put a 4E-width shoe on his foot that was made of soft black leather. It was a walking shoe, a bit athletic-looking, but with suit pants over them the shoes would blend well with his attire.

After stretching the width as much as possible, these shoes were a good option until I could do something better for him. The shoes also came in a size 6E that I could special order for him. That is a **size 13 EEEEEE!!!**

I could take some materials made for soft diabetic insoles and build a cushioning orthotic (arch support) to protect his boney protuberance. It would have a soft gradual sloping form to fit the contours of his feet and protect his relocated arch.

While we were waiting for the new black leather shoes to be delivered, I would see if I could find a store or clinic where Mr. Granby could have his foot molded for custom- made shoes.

The shoe specialty manufacturing company could build his shoes, but it would cost him $1200 and would take over six weeks to get the custom made shoes delivered. How many people with foot problems like his could afford those shoes and wait that long for them?

Mr. Granby had the money and patience, so I helped him schedule an appointment to be molded at an orthopedic shoe store. He was very happy with this solution, but I felt that there had to be many more options out there. I would have to find a way to get the training I needed to find a more medically based job.

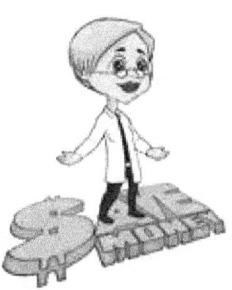

Sharon Carol and her husband, **George**, both had foot and knee problems. They had such a good attitude and made jokes about their pain. In their fifties, they had   stayed in good shape with fitness walks and healthy food.

"Sharon and I have been together so long, we not only look alike, but we have the same pain in the same places!" George chuckled.

"Oh, George, you are such a tease!" Sharon's eyes gleamed.

"Seriously, George and I were having the same painful problems while we were hiking. We were walking on the outside edges of our shoes and wearing them out too fast. Those good athletic shoes aren't cheap, and our ankles and arches were sore.

"We took the time and found an athletic running store that had a special machine and treadmill. The sales person had special training to use a machine to tell us what kind of shoe we should be wearing for our type of feet. We got on this treadmill and a computer recorded our walking footprint. It was all very scientific.

"Yes, and at about the same time, Sharon's and my knees started killing us! My knees never hurt so bad. We haven't been able to walk together for a week now."

I had a suspicion as to what was going on. Hopefully this would be an easy fix.

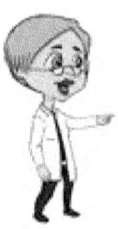

Remember, just because it is a "special store" with "special equipment" doesn't mean that the people running the tests know how to do it correctly or how to analyze the results.

Either ask around in your community of friends and family or ask the person waiting on you how long they have run these tests and whether they have any training certificates. You can also look the store up on the internet and see if anyone has left comments, good or bad, about their service.

Taking off their shoes and socks, I asked Sharon and George to walk for me. They walked away from me; then back toward me slowly, picking up the pace as they normally would. I picked up their new shoes and looked at the sole and heel of each of them.

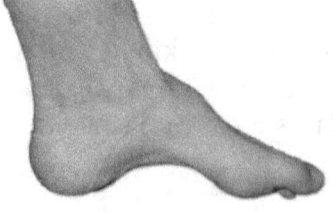

Over Supinator

My suspicions were correct. Both Sharon and George were **over-supinators**. They both walked on the outer edges of their shoes as they had stated. It was more pronounced than I had suspected. Their arches were high and their ankles leaned outward. This kind of arch is called a "cavus" arch. Think of the shape of a cave under the arch.

The problem was that they were wearing shoes for **over-pronators**. That meant that the heel and sole of these special athletic shoes had been built up, or thickened, under the arch side of the feet.

Instead of correcting the feet of a person with over-pronation (flatter arches) the shoes pushed them farther toward the outside edges of their shoes in the direction they were trying to correct; it just aggravated their problems.

I showed them the built-up edges of their shoe soles and what they were doing to their knees. To further illustrate this point, I put a graduated wedge inside their shoes under the outside of the heel. This compensated for the shoe's built up side and made them neutral. Immediately they felt relief.

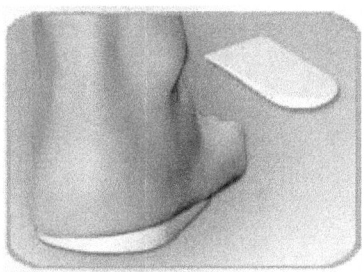

Graduated heel wedge for over-supination

I wrote Sharon and George a note on my pedorthic letter head to take to the runner's shoe store, stating the problem for the shoe clerk to understand. I suggested that they exchange the shoes for those built for an **over-supinator**.

It's a good idea to check on the exchange policy before buying
anything expensive

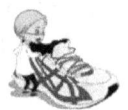

Chapter 3

Journey from Retail to Medical

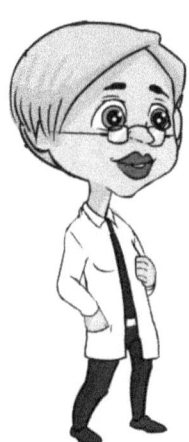

> "'Walk a mile in my shoes' is good advice.' Our children will learn to respect others if they are used to imagining themselves in another's place."
>
> —Rabbi Neil Kurshan

I was surprised by the number of veterans from the local Veteran's Administration clinic who came into our store with brand new custom-orthotics still in their stapled plastic bags.

They came to us in their wheelchairs, crutches, canes, or just walked in wearing their Viet Nam caps or a t-shirt printed with funny or irreverent sayings. I never neglected to thank each one for serving in the military to protect our freedom.

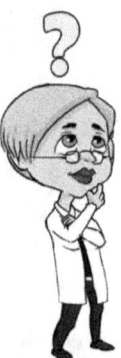

At first I couldn't understand why they would want to have us remake their orthotics for them. The VA clinic paid for the custom-made orthotics that they had brought in to show me.

With permission, I put one of the bright orange orthotics on the floor and stood on it in my stocking feet. Ouch! It was like standing on an orange brick; absolutely no flex or give to them at all.

If I could have spoken with the orthopedic department, I would have tried to help, but who was I to make suggestions when I had no official credentials?

I had been trained by a custom orthotic company. Their representative molded each of the employee's feet for our own custom orthotics. The employees would then practice molding each other's feet with guidance from the DVD given to us by the instructor.

After a period of time, we had to pass a test and were sent a certificate of completion. This enabled us to make custom orthotics with or without a doctor's prescription.

I was able to remake the orthotics for the veterans who came to the store. The new orthotics had a more flexible foundation, which made walking much more comfortable and stable.

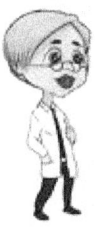 *Many people live every day in their wheel chairs and they may for the rest of their lives. I didn't realize how much a good foot foundation helps them. Whether it is for comfort in their feet or to help keep their leg-joints in line, the right foot support is important for them, too.*

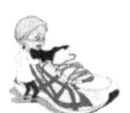

Marianne Smith came to the shoe store on a beautiful day in May. She was a young lawyer and a little "closed and tight" in conversation in the beginning. She didn't believe anyone could help her and felt bitter about promises that others had made to her about her feet.

After some warm-up conversation, she finally let go of her defensiveness and spoke candidly.

"What was the beginning of your feet getting into this shape? How long have you had to suffer this way?" I asked.

"I was in gymnastics as a child. Before I turned eleven, I was in constant practice for competition vaulting. Being gifted, my parents ignored the doctor's warnings and encouraged me to work harder, and train longer. I try not to blame them, but I can hardly walk with the pain anymore."

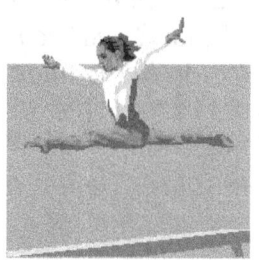

Gymnastics competition

Since her bones were still forming as a child; the constant abuse left her nearly crippled as an adult. She had experienced many surgeries, but some harmed her more than helped her. (*Unfortunately I had heard statements like this a lot about certain types of foot surgeries*)

In this case, she didn't need more control of her arches and foot joints; she needed less control with more padding and support. This is called an **accommodative** type of support.

I used her feet as a template and hand-made a pair of firm, but soft supports inside a pair of Rocker Bottom shoes. In this case, the shoes turned out to be just the right answer.

Now her feet wouldn't drop down solidly on the heels and balls of her feet. They would be continuously cushioned, and the rocker bottom would allow her to roll her feet from heel to toe instead of pushing off with her big toe. She wouldn't have the impact on her bones that she would have in regular flat-bottom shoes.

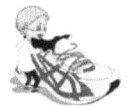

Back to School!

With these kinds of customers in need, I decided to go back to school at the shoe store's **Certified Pedorthic training** in their South Eastern headquarters located in Atlanta, Georgia.

On the way to my first class the orange blossoms fell like snowflakes. The air was warm, humid and sweet. I had waited so long for this day. Soon, I would be able to help the people who came to me with a more professional, medical knowledge.

I learned a lot about the anatomy and problems of the feet and how the problems would affect the rest of the body.

It was interesting to see where and how the custom orthotics were manufactured from the molds I had shipped to them. Much of the hands-on learning was from the practice the students did on each other's feet after the instruction.

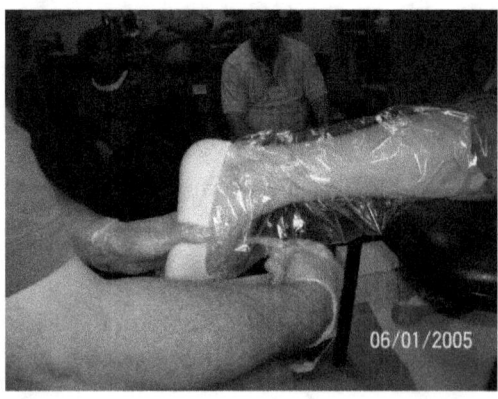

06/01/2005

Students practicing molding feet for orthotics

After weeks of full-time training, it was back to the shoe store where I worked in Denver. This was the time for more on-the-job practice of all I had learned. The certification required the trainee to log 1000 hours working and practicing before taking an all-day test.

At the appointed time I went to the testing facility at the Auraria College Campus, located in Denver, Colorado. My brain was fried after the testing. I couldn't do anything but rest for a while. The hardest part was the waiting the two *loooooong* months to find out if I had passed.

The day I got the letter of acceptance, my husband and I stepped out of the car in the middle of the street and did the "happy dance" together beside the mailboxes.

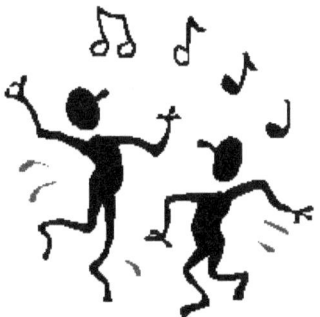

Happy Dance!

I began studying magazines that catered to the *Orthopedic and Prosthetic Professional*. In the back of the magazines was a section about employment and often articles about specific companies.

One company caught my attention each time I looked at the magazine, but there were no openings in my geographical area. One day a few months later, I was scanning the ads as usual and froze. I reread the ad about six more times before I could believe what I was seeing.

The Medical O & P facility that had my attention was looking for a Certified Pedorthist about thirteen miles from my home.

When I called the district manager at the Facility, I was told that they were looking for someone who had more experience working in a medical setting than I had. I wanted to work at this Medical O & P facility and I wasn't giving up.

No one the company had interviewed wanted that location. The manager had even flown someone in from Oklahoma.

The Medical O&P office and orthopedic shoe store had never made a profit at this location and the district manager was willing to try something different to increase their sales. Since I had been working in retail, they felt I might become an asset.

As I drove around the neighborhood of the store, I saw that we could show the community we were just around the corner waiting to make their lives better.

Using several gallons of paint and restocking all the walls with product would go a long way toward improving the store's inviting appearance.

Upon presenting this vision to the district and regional managers, they decided to give me a try. I had passion. Believing I could make a difference, I was hired as a certified pedorthist at an hourly wage, on trial.

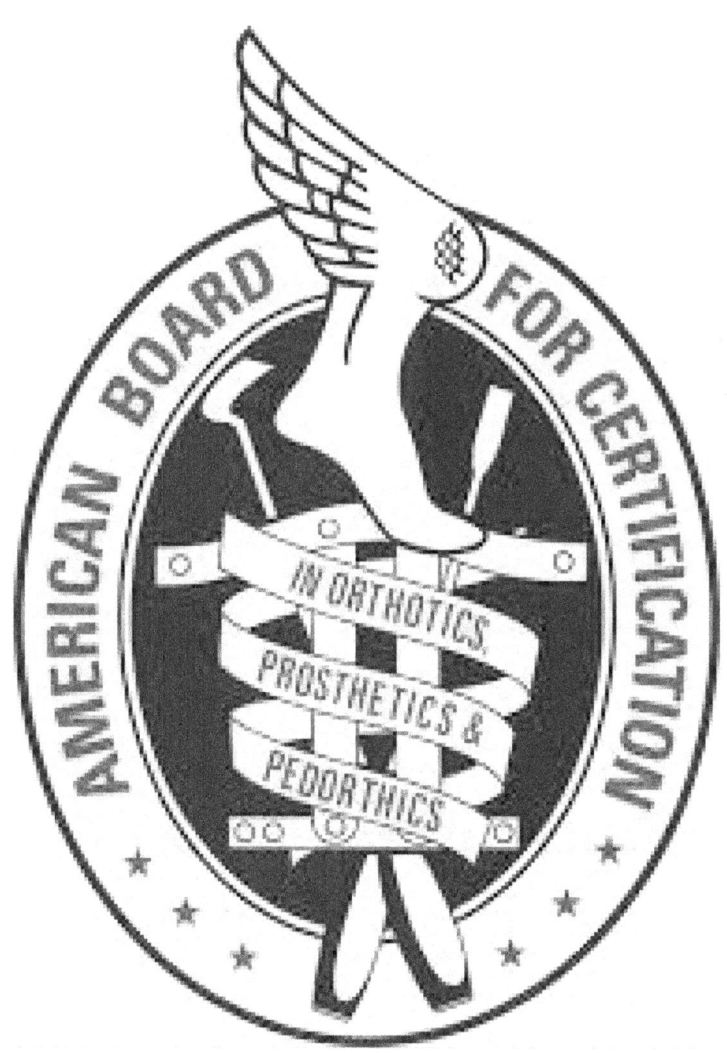

ABC Credentials from the Orthopedic/Prosthetic Certifying Association

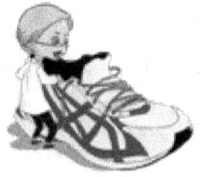

Caution

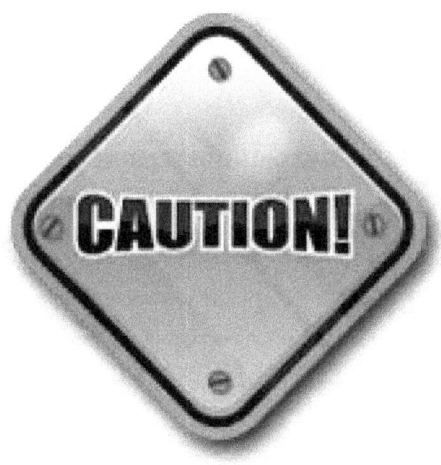

The next section has graphic content
(maybe intense for weak stomachs)

My initiation into the hard-core medical side of this profession was a stomach turner. I was sent to accompany another certified pedorthist and an orthopedic surgeon on hospital rounds. The encounter brought to light what I would be dealing with on a normal day while working at the orthopedic shoe store.

As the physician spoke to the patient, a man in his fifties, he removed the blood-soaked bandages on a wound so deep and large I could see the muscles, veins, tendons, and all the way to the bone.

The doctor decided the wound needed to be *abraded* (dead flesh cut away) so that the fresher flesh would have more blood flow to heal.

Watching him take the "Dremel-type" electrical tool and grind away inside that hole while the patient sat and talked as if nothing were happening, was a very shocking experience!

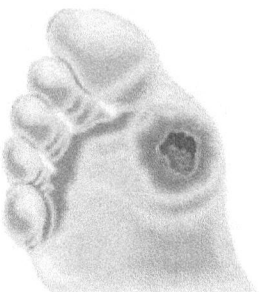

Foot ulcer

The patient had severe **neuropathy** from diabetes that had destroyed nerve sensation in his lower extremities. He could no longer feel exterior pain, but had a constant phantom sensation of his legs and feet "going to sleep."

(Not all neuropathy is a side effect of diabetes. There can be injury, illness, and other reasons a patient would develop neuropathy.)

I passed the first test. I didn't throw-up on the doctor's shoes. My stomach flew up and down like I had my own personal roller coaster, flipped over, and fought hard to come out my throat.

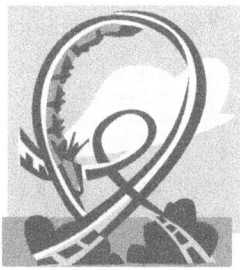

Roller coaster stomach

The next patient that same day was a Latin American man in his forties. He was recovering from the fourteenth surgery on his feet. Having surgery again and again as each toe had been amputated, eventually he also lost portions of his feet. Finally his legs ended at his ankles.

Skin had been gathered and sewn together to leave as much padding as possible at the end of his ankles so he could try to stand if he had prosthetic feet. I not only had to get used to the sights and smells of freshly healing flesh, but felt empathy for the enormous losses these people had suffered.

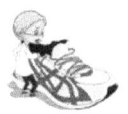

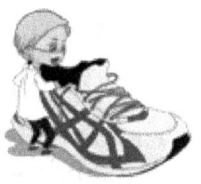

Chapter 4

Amputations and Suicide

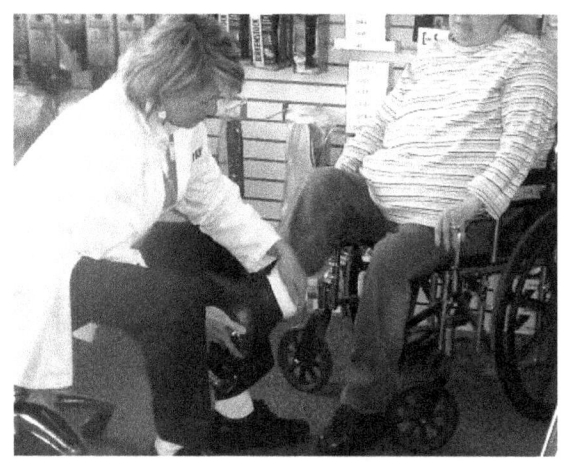

"I had the blues because I had no shoes until upon the street, I met a man who had no feet."

—Denis Waitley, Motivational Author/Speaker

Javier Gonzales was wheeled into my examination room. He was the patient I had met on my last hospital visit, who had lost both his feet. Javier was joined by his warm and friendly wife, Maria and his second son of five, Carlos.

It was obvious the family had great love for each other and concern for Javier's future. Javier was very depressed. His wife spoke up to explain the history of Javier's despair.

"Javier is only forty-five. He used to play competition pool, and we loved to dance.
He is a hard worker and feels very bad about not earning money at a job. For two years they kept taking him to surgery. Finally the surgeries stopped when his feet were gone."

"Maria, why wasn't Javier fitted for prosthetic feet? He is a healthy young man with many years ahead and the prosthetics are very good now. "

"The doctors told us he would never walk again without fitted prosthetic feet, which we cannot afford. His insurance ended when he lost his job. He has been in that wheelchair for three years now."

Javier's future looked dismal. I felt very sorry as I looked at the emptiness of his missing feet.

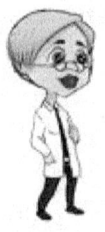 *Most of the amputations I saw were caused by unchecked diabetes. Diabetes constricts the vascular system at the outer extremities first. The heart has to make a stronger effort to pump the blood through the veins and arteries; this is another reason diabetes is associated with heart disease. Bit by bit, as the extremity flesh dies from*

lack of oxygen and nutrients, that portion must be removed to save the rest of the foot.

Javier wanted to find a shoe "looking" devise to stay on the end of his ankles. He needed something to help him look normal and keep him warmer in the cold winter months ahead. He never planned to walk again.

I had other plans for him!

A high percentage of my clients were over seventy. Often the spouse would come to see me after their loved one passed away. Sometimes they would bring a pair of shoes that had never been worn before the death. It made them feel better to bring the shoes to my "donation box." There were a few charities in the area of the store that my office would contribute to with these shoes.

In the donation box, I found a pair of shoes with an opening that I thought I could tighten around Javier's ankles. I sent the family home with the shoes, a new appointment, and an idea for a new beginning.

While contemplating the next appointment I would have with Javier, there were three more patients waiting to be seen before the day was done. Wishing I could have drawn out my plans for Javier, I would have to be content looking at my notes later and designing my ideas for him.

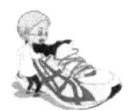

My office assistant led **Nancy Seville** to the door of the exam room. I directed Nancy and her son, Mark, to be seated. Looking at her file I saw who had examined her last. The employee who had worked at this office just before I was hired had worked with Nancy.

"I swore I would never come back to this place, but my son made me."

"Why is that, Nancy, what was the problem?"
"That man scared me and made me feel bad."

"Can you tell me about your experience last year, Nancy?"

"I tried to tell him these ugly shoes are too big, I kept falling on the stairs. He wouldn't listen to me. When I spoke up about it, he yelled at me and kept stuffing more liners in the shoes to try and make them fit. I finally kept my mouth shut and cried when I got home."

"I'm sorry to hear you had a bad experience. What can I do to make you feel better now?"

"It doesn't matter; I am going to commit suicide next week." She looked straight into my eyes.

"Why, Nancy?"

"No one cares, no one listens to me. I have pain and I feel ugly and terrible."

Instinctively I reached out and gave her a hug. She stayed in the hug and began to cry, then to sob. Heart wrenching sounds came from her slight body.

"Nancy, if your feet felt better and you thought your shoes look pretty, would that help any?"

"The other shoe man said these were the only choices I had. Black or white and orthopedic; they look like an old man's shoes. I know people stare at them and there is not one thing I can wear with them.

"You would just be wasting your time at 'looks good.' I hate them, but I have no other choice for these painful, ugly feet of mine."

"Well Nancy, would you trust me long enough to let me show you some other possibilities? I think some more choices are available to you now." Her eyes were wide; then narrowed in doubt.

"I don't want to get my hopes up like the last time."

"I will be right back. Do you need a cup of water and a Kleenex?" She nodded slowly.

I listened to her talk about her children who lived far away, and how she missed a friend who had died recently.

While I "heard" more than her words, I measured her feet and wrote the numbers in the chart, noticing the bony bunions at the sides of her feet (a painful swelling on the first joint of the big toe).

"Nancy, I am going to bring a few choices for you and we will go over why each of these would be good for your feet, OK?"

I quickly went to my stockroom and had my fingers crossed that the shoes I thought would be perfect for her were available in her size.

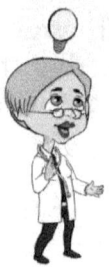

Bingo! You could tell from her clothes that she liked red, and she had some cheaply made brown shoes that gave her no support at all. But she obviously liked brown, as her purse was that color, too.

The red leather shoes I had in mind for her had a pretty floral design cut in the leather at the toe and two Velcro strap fasteners. With the arthritis in her hands I knew these would be easier for her to fasten.

There were two different styles of medium-brown shoes. One had shoe strings, but I could use elastic shoe strings and she would not have to tie them. The brown ones had a t-strap closure. They still held the foot in place, but looked dressy.

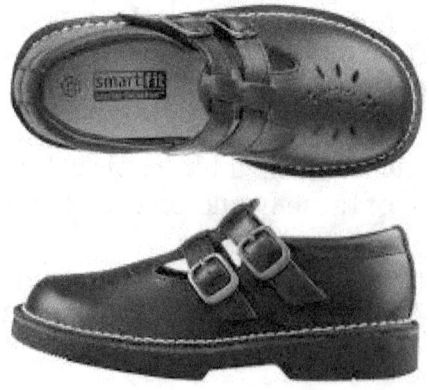

Nancy's new shoes

48

"Nancy, let's try these on. We have a full length mirror over here were you can look at yourself."

She was like a kid in a candy store. Red jaw-breaker shoes and chocolate brown strap shoes; which would be her favorites?

"I love these dressy brown ones, but they are a little tight at the side of my big toe."

"Not a problem, Nancy. There is a special tool just for that. When you decide if that is really your favorite, I will stretch them for you."

We tried on the others, but came back to those brown ones. "So, when can you stretch them? Can I get them next week?"

It was amazing how her attitude had changed. She sounded and looked like a different person.

"You can wait right there, Nancy, and I will bring them back for you to try on again."

I took them to the work bench where the shoe and bunion stretchers were kept. Spraying the inside and outside with an alcohol based fluid, I inserted the bunion tool. This is a metal ball mounted on a tool that looks like something you might use to shoe a horse.

On the opposite side of the tool was a ring that the ball would fit through when the tool was closed. With long handles, I could get a good pressure with the side of her shoe in-between the ball and ring.

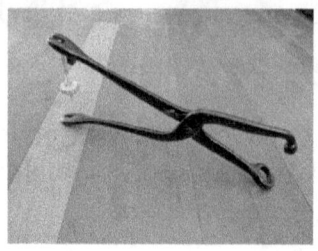

Ball and ring bunion stretcher

As I held this tool in place, I took my heat gun (*looks like a VERY hot blow dryer*) and circled hot air inside and outside of the shoe. When I took the tool out, there was a "bubble" created along the big toe side of the shoe and now she had a pocket in the leather for her bunion to fit just right.

I smoothed the leather a little so it didn't look obvious. Nancy was waiting expectantly in the exam room, where I placed the shoes on her feet as if she were Cinderella. I knew she needed to feel special. They fit perfectly.

"Oh, they feel great! See, I can walk around and don't feel that awful pain. They look pretty. My neighbor friends will like them too, and I can wear them with a dress or pants. I can't believe it. I thought I had to wear ugly shoes forever."

I instructed Nancy and her son on the "break-in period" of the new shoes so as not to cause any blisters or callouses. Then I explained to them both that Nancy should examine her feet EVERY evening to make sure she could see any red pressure points developing. They were to let me know right away if that were the case.

After Nancy paid, she put her old shoes in the box and wore the new ones out. I got another hug at the door and many thanks from Nancy as well as her son.

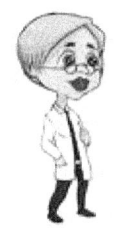

Nancy had diabetes and other medical symptoms that enabled her to get a pair of approved shoes and diabetic inserts once a year. For an entire year, these would probably be the only shoes she wore, day in and day out.

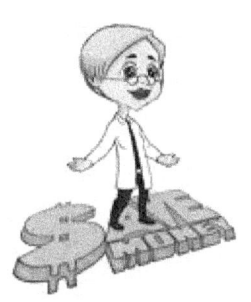

I would always suggest buying a second pair so the first pair could dry out and "rebound" from being compressed all day. This would make both pair of shoes last longer. I gave a 10% discount for the second pair to encourage the purchase.

Many people with diabetes have neuropathy as a secondary condition. Neuropathy constricts the blood flow to the outer extremities and damages the nerve endings. Nancy might not feel it if she had dropped a bottle cap in her shoe, which could cause a deep, bottle-cap-shaped wound, nor would she be able to tell if she was getting a bad, bloody blister.

This is what it is all about for me. Listening is the biggest part of the service in my opinion. Paying attention to patients' concerns, needs, style, color preference, and economic level helps me steer them to a good option. Keeping in touch and checking up on them when they have a condition that could cause further complications is also very important.

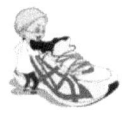

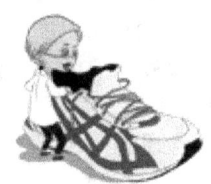

Chapter 5

Prickles to Prisoners

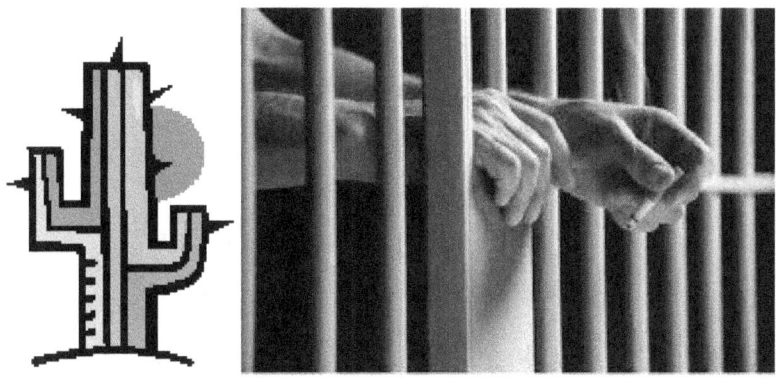

"A lie can travel halfway around the world while the truth is putting on its shoes." —Charles Spurgeon

Anne Prickle: Boy howdy, she lived up to her name!

The first time I saw Anne, I saw a small, older woman talking at the top of her lungs into her cell phone. My waiting room was completely full when I came from the exam room. The other clients were disturbed by her loud rudeness.

She had come for her appointment thirty minutes too early and was already on the phone to Kaiser HMO to say she was being ignored and mistreated. My office assistant had already reminded her of the time of her appointment, but she kept on complaining to Kaiser. I moved her into the examination room to calm the other patients.

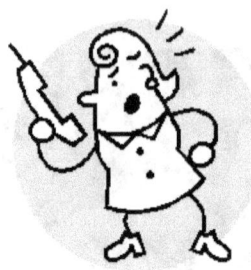

Complaining loudly on the phone

Kaiser HMO called our office to find out what was going on. I explained the situation, and they told me it had happened before with other offices she had been to. It was an ominous warning.

Anne felt that everyone abused her, ignored her, and belittled her. She complained about her children, siblings, doctors, bus drivers, etc....I don't think anyone was exempt. She felt if she complained loudly enough she would always get her way; it had worked many times before.

Another kind client offered his own appointment to get Anne out of the store faster. I thanked him and went in to find out what Anne needed. I tried everything. I was sweet, nice, kind, tried to sympathize, empathize, but nothing worked.

She told me the doctor wanted her to wear "box toe shoes" I brought multiple pairs in this style. They had a deeper toe box, commonly used to give more room for bunions or hammer toes. She hated them all because she thought they were too heavy, but more importantly, she believed her friends would laugh at her. Then I found a lighter weight shoe in a darker color so they would look smaller.

She was satisfied until she wore them to a luncheon with her friends and someone said she looked ridiculous.

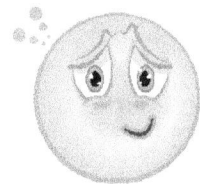

Embarrassed by friends

Back she came, calling Kaiser and complaining again as we did not "get it right" the first time. Louder and more obnoxious she became. Let me tell you now, the customer is NOT always right!

I settled her in the exam room and looked her in the eyes. She had been verbally abusive to me and my staff as well as annoying the other clients.

"Anne, this is not acceptable behavior from you. If you don't stop this behavior, you will have to leave. I would be happy to help you if you will calm down and work with us"

She looked at me with some surprise and was quiet for a few minutes. Then I could tell she was testing me to see if I was "for real."

Yes, I was!

She treated me with more respect for a while. But that was not the end of it. She reverted several times to her old ways and had to be reminded each time.

Finally, she continued to bring shoes back and wanted refunds even when she had approved them and I had modified them for her feet. I told Kaiser I thought she might be happier working with someone else.

The Kaiser counselors said she had been through all of them and no one could handle her. I told them I was sorry, but I could not counsel her and tolerate the abuse for my establishment any longer. She was blocked.

About two weeks later she came in asking to be let back in as a client. I was cordial and gave her alternate suggestions, but **every patient was important and deserved to have peace and consideration in my facility.**

I wished her well, but believe I made the right decision.

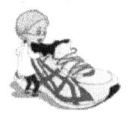

My first meeting with **Carl Black** included a uniformed prison guard who accompanied him into my office. Complete with his day-stick and gun, Carl's guard watched every move he made.

"This is my body guard. Wouldn't want you puttin' the moves on me! Now I wouldn't mind that, but my friend here might get jealous."

I brushed Carl's hand away as he reached swiftly for my knee.

Carl wore a bright orange jump-suit with the words "Department of Corrections" stenciled in big black letters on his back.

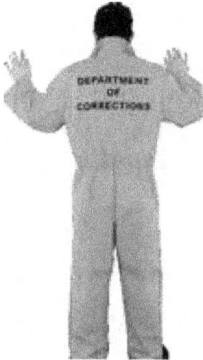

County prisoner

This is not a good way to take care of your foot pain on a budget! The county government paid for his treatment.

While I took Carl's shoes off, he tried to look down my blouse as he excitedly explained why he was in jail.

"I met some real high-rollers this time. We were drinking all night and I had a chick on both sides for luck. It was all worth it. I would do it again in a minute, but I didn't start the fight that landed me in prison and if the knife had just been a quarter inch to the left...oh well, what can I say?" Carl tried to look innocent and shrugged his shoulders.

I saw that Carl had an amputation with fresh surgery on his left foot (a 'Liz Frank' amputation) cut off at the mid-arch. There were several bandages layered around his foot, and I knew the doctor expected me to un-wrap the sterile bandage, cover the wound with sterile plastic wrap, and not cause Carl any more problems. This would allow me to carefully measure his foot and decide on appropriate footwear. No fresh infection while in my examination room!

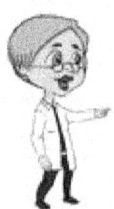
Be your own doctor and watch out for yourself. When you have any open wounds on your feet, just like in a restaurant, don't let anyone touch your wound if they have sneezed and caught it or handled something and didn't put their examination gloves on. It should be a fresh pair from a box of disposables for each patient.

Carl calmed down and got more serious as I showed real concern for him and his foot problems.

"Last time I was here, the other shoe doctor gave me these shoes. I have had a hard time keeping them on with half my foot missing and I believe these shoes are what started my new ulcer."

Uh-oh! I excused myself and talked with the district manager by phone. You see, I agreed with him.

The shoes he wore into the store were too big for him and were not high-tops. There was no way for him to be comfortable or to keep them secure around his ankle. I was aghast! The constant rubbing on his skin from the shoe was the worst situation for a person with diabetes and neuropathy.

The former employee had been dismissed so I could not discuss the situation with him. I knew Carl needed my help and I would do my best.

Molding his feet for custom-made shoes, I realized Carl would be getting out of jail before the pair would come back from manufacturing. Normally the correctional facility would pay for his shoes, but I knew Carl could not afford them. There was nothing to do but absorb the cost and do the right thing by Carl.

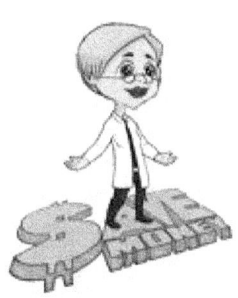

Don't be deceived; these "helping humans with compassion" businesses are still a business. There are very good people employed in these places, but all of them, ultimately, have to consider the bottom line and report what they spend to their bosses.

Carl and I worked together with his medical doctor for many months before I really felt he was safe. It took six weeks for his shoes to come back to the store.

At Carl's next appointment it was time to smooth the edges and make sure his toe fillers and cushioned orthotics fit correctly. No sharp edges or ledges around and under his feet. I gave him break-in instructions and saw him periodically for the next few weeks to make sure everything was working properly and his doctor was satisfied.

Carl stopped putting the moves on me and treated me politely as a professional. Now, any other woman working in the office was still fair game!

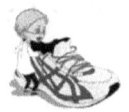

Chapter 6

Stand Alone

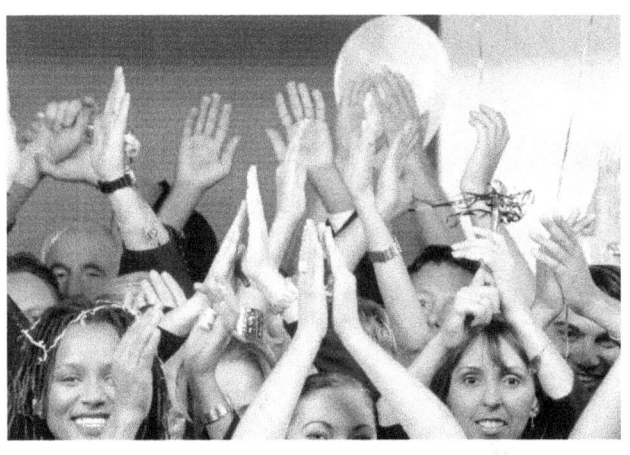

"Our wounds are often the openings in to the best and most beautiful part of us." —*David Richo*

It was time to help **Javier Gonzales** get on with his life. The following Monday morning, I prepared the pre-plastered strips of cloth, a Styrofoam molding box, surgical scissors, plastic bags, blue marking pen, measuring tape, bucket of water, forms, and floor protectant for Javier's appointment.

"Are you doing OK today, Javier?"

"I'm as well as can be expected."

"Well let's get busy, OK?"

With the floor protected and gloves on my hands, I dipped the plaster strips in water one by one. When they were soaked through, I brought the strips out to wrap Javier's ankles and lower legs.

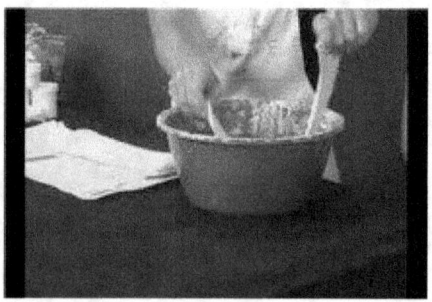

Preparing wet plaster strips

As the plaster hardened, it created a shell. I marked the sides and front of the cast so there would be no mistaking which was the front and back of the mold. Then, with special medical scissors, I cut down the front of the molds and eased his ankles and calves out.

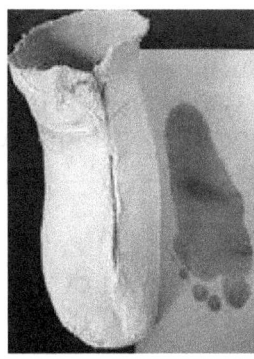

Plaster cast, cut and removed

I pushed the ends of his legs into the Styrofoam box and took photographs. Each three-dimensional picture I could create for the shoe and insert manufacturer would help get an exact fit. It was very different working without an arch, ball of foot, or a heel to reference. The measurements and information needed were written on a form and include with the molds.

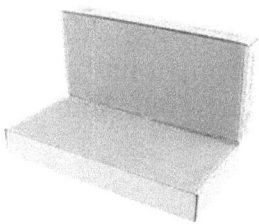

Foam molding box for impressions of the end of Javier's ankles

Now I could get off the floor and my 15-inch shoe-fitting stool. Whew!

Then the fun part began. I worked to get the Gonzales family to participate in choosing style, color, and materials. If I could get them involved, they would become more invested in the project and could look forward to something that was not so "orthopedic" looking.

In Javier's case, high-top shoes were a necessity as they would tighten around his ankles and lower calves. He liked the athletic look and dressed youthfully. I found a company that would let me choose colors and textures outside of the normal black and white leather choices.

The shoes needed to be shorter than he would have normally worn as we didn't want the front of the toe to bend and throw him forward on his face.

I gave the company the measurements and molds, the kind of padding inside the shoes that was required for Javier's sensitive skin, and then I decided on the dense foam inserts to cushion and hold the ankles and bottom of his leg ends in position.

It would take six weeks for the molds to be shipped and the shoes to return to me. Fortunately the shoe company hurried a bit on this one and we got them back in four weeks.

For the first time, Javier and his wife looked excited and expectant. This appointment had a decidedly different mood. I settled him in the exam room and brought in the large shoe box with me.

Taking Javier's new "basketball" style shoes from the box, there were smiles around the room. The shoes were a mesh and leather blend just like any other athletic style. There was even a shoe logo of their company impressed in the leather!

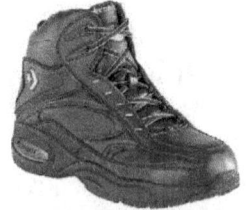

Javier's new custom athletic shoe

I had to see how they would fit: that there were no gaps and that they would not rub certain spots as the shoe shifted and bent. I had to remember that Javier had serious diabetes. I didn't want him to lose anything else due to an irritation that could cause an ulcer.

Inside the front of the foot where the toes should be was the "toe filler." This was dense foam attached to the liner under his ankle. I then added a poly carbon plate under his liner so the shoe would hardly bend, but would still have spring to help propel him forward over the toe area.

I gave instructions to Javier's wife, Maria, to watch for red pressure marks. There was a "break-in" schedule for how long he should wear the shoes and liners each day. As he got used to them, he could increase the wear time and I would alter it as necessary.

Things worked fine for a few days, but as Javier stood and tried to walk more aggressively, balancing with his cane, the shoe on the smaller ankle would turn around on his foot until the toe of the shoe was coming out to the side. I was happy to see his confidence rising, but we had to commence the "Taming of the Shoe."

I asked an orthotics brace-maker to give her opinion about Javier's situation. She was one of the best in the field and her clients loved her. I was lucky to have her as a friend and co-worker.

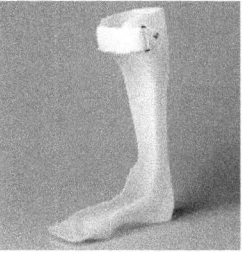

Plastic AFO brace

We determined that an AFO (under the foot, around the calf, plastic brace) could be inserted into Javier's shoe and would hold the toe of the shoe in the front and straight forward.

Javier no longer needs a wheelchair for his mobility. He has gained back his participation in most of the activities he enjoyed in the past. The Medical O & P company printed the story about Javier with a picture in their yearly calendar. Carlos and Javier's other children decided to put on a dinner dance to raise money for the cost of Javier's brace and shoes. All their friends and family were invited to bring donations as they enjoyed the celebration.

The day of the dance, Javier was wheeled into the room. Everyone got very quiet as the music started and Javier stood and danced with his wife, Maria. The friends and family gave them a standing ovation and there wasn't a dry eye in the house.

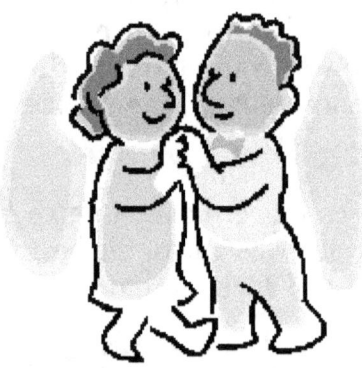

Chapter 7

All You Need is Love!

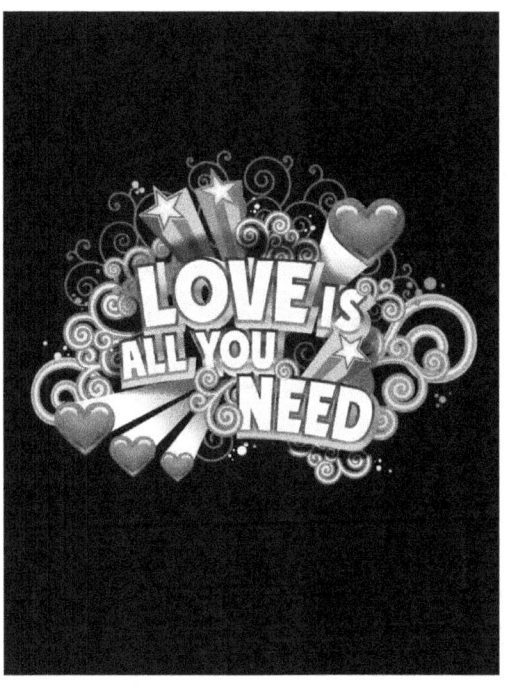

"I met in the street a very poor young man who was in love. His hat was old, his coat worn, his cloak was out at the elbows, the water passed through his shoes, - and the stars through his soul."
—Victor Hugo

"Hooray!"

Five minutes after closing, the rest of my staff had left the store, except for Ken, the orthopedic manager in the connected offices.

The quiet and solitude always helped me think as I settled at my desk to catch up and plan the next day's work.

The front entrance door was locked and the outer lights turned off. I grabbed my Diet Pepsi from the 'fridge and a leftover donut stuck to the bottom of the bakery box.

In the silence I heard footsteps and Ken with another man rounded the wall to my office.

"Lynda, this is Mr. Ryder. He was asked to visit you by Dr. Kuttz at the Golden Clinic. He waited on our side of the building for an hour; a misunderstanding with the office ladies."

"Ken, all my employees have gone home."

"Don't worry; if you can take care of Mr. Ryder, I will be here for another hour."

Mr. Ryder's eyes were NOT pleading with me to stay and take care of him. As he spoke he looked angry.

"I see you don't have any time for me. Just give me what I had last year like *he* always does."

The "he" Mr. Ryder referred to was the former employee, who had worked in my position. The truth is, if it really was his way of doing business, Medicare, the doctor, and Mr. Ryder would have grounds to pursue actions against the Medical O&P Company.

68

"Mr. Ryder, we will make time right now to examine your feet properly. A lot of changes happen throughout our bodies in a year."

"No, no...I don't want it. Forget it, I'm leaving!"

"Mr. Ryder, can we look at your file together?" He glared at me as he sat down.

In an orthopedic store, information must be recorded in the patient's file. The doctor's prescription and insurance information taken by the administrative assistant: important facts about the patient's size, weight, occupation, style and color preferences, all must be included.

The certified pedorthist records sizes, shapes, abnormal callouses, pressure points, ulcers, amputations; any abnormality of the foot, ankle, skin conditions, lower leg swelling, redness, etc....

Any program of ambulation, wound healing, or change in major issues, must be recorded in the patient's file. If the patient is non-compliant with the protective program the physician has outlined, they must be reported to the physician or nurse practitioner involved in the case.

"Ok, have you gotten this same shoe style each year? Are you having pain in your feet anywhere?"

As I continued to ask him questions, he seemed to relax a bit. I began to touch his shoes as I pointed out areas that I questioned.

Leading him to the examination room, I kept eye contact with Mr. Ryder while untying and slipping his shoes and socks off.

The smell was incredible. Not the frequent "haven't-changed-socks-in-a-week" smell; this was a "something-is-dead, rotting, needs-to-be-buried" smell.

Some pieces of Mr. Ryder's skin were stuck to his socks and some were falling on the pad I had put under his feet. Due to diabetes and the resulting neuropathy, Mr. Ryder's feet were numb and he had little circulation in them. The flesh was dying. He watched for my reaction.

My job was to observe, record and notify the doctor or foot health nurse of redness, very warm areas, oozing and open callouses or blisters, swelling, anything that was already a limb threatening problem or a situation that could develop into one.

There were specific tests for the degree of neuropathy or insensitivity in his feet, temperature, leg length discrepancy, and measurements that had to be recorded. The plan of action was in the file where all those involved could easily check on the progress.

Thinking fast before gagging and coughing, I excused myself, telling him I had to make a quick phone call. I ran around the corner and found the *Vicks VapoRub* stashed for just such an occasion.

Wiping some of the Vicks under each of my nostrils, I breathed deeply, grabbed a cup of water for each of us, and returned to Mr. Ryder.

My responsibility was to accurately record and report the examination and my findings to the physician treating Mr. Ryder. Each year he was eligible for another pair of diabetic approved shoes and two pair of diabetic inserts as long as his insurance still approved them and the physician treating him still verified his diabetic and neuropathic condition.

We talked about topics that interested Mr. Ryder, especially trout fishing. Continuing to measure and examine his feet I put his socks and shoes back on during the conversation.

All that I had observed was recoded in his file and I would contact his physician the following day.

Mr. Ryder paused, straightened and stared into my eyes, nodding slightly. His eyes were moist and wide.

"Thank you."

"You're Welcome."

Pride intact, Mr. Ryder shook my hand and said he looked forward to our next appointment.

One day someone will do the same for someone in my family.

All you need is love...

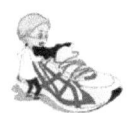

I used sign language. No, I don't know real sign language; maybe more like body language.

A beautiful Latin American family came into the store one afternoon: a mother, dad, and five children. The mother looked very tired. She was a petite woman and I could tell her husband was feeling protective of her.

Having lived in other countries, I knew how hard it could be to get someone to understand you when you don't know their culture, customs, and language. Sometimes it's frustrating, and can make people feel nervous and anxious.

This family was young so even the children were afraid to talk, though they knew a few English words. All I could tell was that there was a problem and it was about the mother.

I sat on my Harley Davidson motorcycle seat that was a stool with wheels. My husband, Roque had found it for my birthday and I used it every day at the store. The children liked it when I backed up and said, "Beep, beep, beep." I wanted to make them smile and feel more comfortable.

'*Familia*' sounded like a word they knew, '*Madre*' for mother and '*zapatos*' meaning shoes. OK; that was about my limit of spanish words. From there we improvised.

I picked up *Madre's* foot, pointed to it then shrugged. The husband and wife talked it over with the eldest child, until *Madre* pointed to the bottom of her foot and toes.

She proceeded to show me actions of washing clothes in pantomime and the husband said a word that sounded like 'hospital'. I think they were telling me she washed clothes in the hospital and she was on her feet all day. Evidently, *Padre* had not found a job yet and watched after the children and the house where they were staying.

Madre was wearing some very thin loafer-type shoes. Ugh! Just looking at them made my feet hurt. I had to figure out how to help her "on the cheap" as he was taking out his wallet to show me how much money they could afford. It was about the amount of a McDonald's Happy Meal.

This lady needed new supportive shoes but couldn't afford them, but I could do something to help. I looked around the store for more cushion and support to put under her feet.

Holding her shoe, I showed them I was going to tear out her glued-in liners. They were not impressed. *Padre* was not sure about this and looked skeptical. I just smiled and waited. *Madre* was really hurting, so she was ready to take a chance on me.

I did it quickly, like taking a Band-Aid off before the victim knows what hit them. Of course, you don't let them see under the Band-Aid before you cover the wound!

Carrying her shoes into the store room, I remembered that we had changed manufacturers on a line of orthotics. We had a few left I that was planning to put out on the mark-down shelf.

I was able to cut the arch supports to the right size using her shoe liner as a pattern. I measured the arch against her foot to make sure the arch fit her in the right place. She would need more support than this, but this was a start.

The children all stayed right in their seats and listened to their parents. It was really refreshing to see this. This was often not what I experienced with other clients' children. Giving all the children a Tootsie Roll, I asked them not to unwrap them until they were outside.

Keeping leftover pieces of Poron and PPT (thin, dense cushion materials) I was able to fashion a more graduated arch and glue it onto the support that I had cut to size.

As I lifted her foot and removed her socks, I saw red calloused spots under the balls of her foot and heel. The metatarsal heads at the base of her toes had pressured against the floor through the thin shoes. This was causing her a lot of pain when standing and walking.

Taping pieces of cotton to her sock where the pressure spots were located, I put lipstick on each of the cotton pieces. She then stood in her shoe. With her foot out of her shoes, I could tell exactly where I needed to give her relief on the arch supports. We repeated the process on the other foot.

After turning the arch supports over, I ground out the spots where the lipstick had marked the arch supports and filled them with a much softer gel material. Then I put a graduated pad (metatarsal pad) behind the pressure spots so it would offload those sore, red places even more.

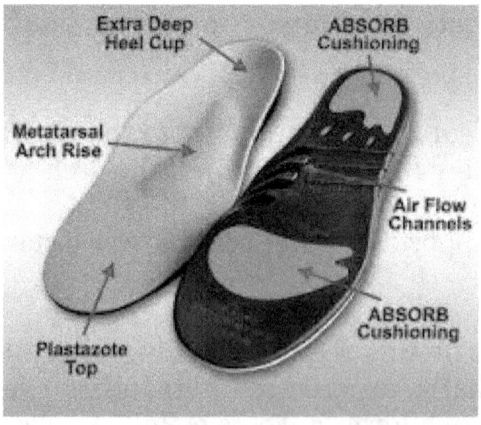

Arch supports with metatarsal pads.

It was time for her to try the new arch supports in her shoes. If I had not taken the original inserts out, the new arch supports would have made her shoes too tight. I waited and watched as she walked across the room.

Madre smiled and clapped her hands. *Padre* and the children nodded and laughed. It was not a complete answer for her, but it was a beginning of trust.

I showed them some shoes with shoe strings that would give her much more support and they were a more casual, athletic type shoe that would really hug the arch and have more cushioning in the sole.

Padre showed me his wallet and I knew he wanted to know how much they would cost. I wrote down the amount. I also knew the word "*dinero,*" so he nodded his head, "yes."

One month later they were back. *Padre* was so proud and happy he had earned the money for *Madre's* shoes himself. He was probably doing some house painting, by the look of his pants and shirt.

I took *Madre's* shoes off her feet and slipped the arch supports I had constructed into the new shoes. As she walked back and forth on the carpet, I motioned for her to try them out on the concrete. Hesitantly all seven of them filed out into the bright sunlight.

Padre came in alone about fifteen minutes later and pushed the money into my palm as he shook my hand.

It is hard to let people go out like that without more instructions, without talking about the warranty and telling them to come back if they have problems, but I think they knew that I would still be there for them.

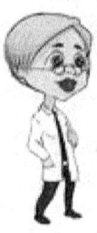

If Madre were a diabetic, had open sores, looked like there were any other problems, I would have waited until I could find someone to interpret. I could not have treated the sale as a retail purchase if Madre had handed me a doctor's prescription.

I dealt with many nationalities in the store. Sometimes there were children or grandchildren to help. A few times I called my husband, Roque, who speaks spanish and Italian. He enjoyed helping Italian speakers, as the younger generations frequently do not speak their ancestral language.

(My husband is from Lima, Peru. I am a lucky woman. **Viva el Peru**!)

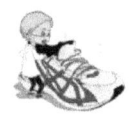

Italy is known for some of the best made, most expensive, most beautiful shoes in the world. After all, the country is shaped like a boot!

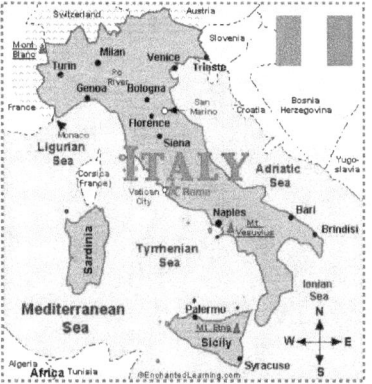

Italian "boot"

Italian shoes are normally made on a narrow *last*. (*This is a shoe-shaped form to stretch the leather on as the shoes are constructed.*) The German shoe is normally made on a wider *last* for the culturally wider German foot.

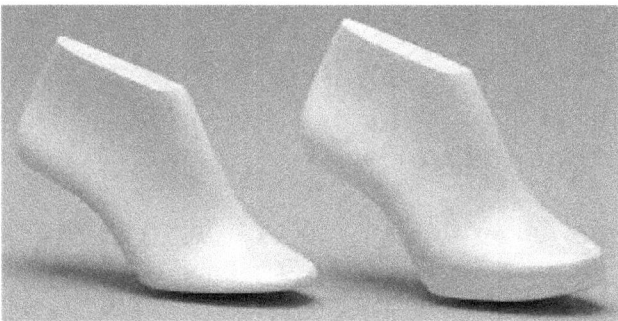

Shoe "last"

Many older Italian women have an image identity connected to the shape and size of their shoes. Style is very important.

Many women of any nationality are in denial about their shoe size and have walked out of shoe stores upset when shown their true shoe size. Even looking down and seeing the size for themselves; they believe the measuring device is either broken or the sales clerk is demented!

Sophia was a favorite customer of mine because of her spirit, not because she was easy to work with or a compliant patient for her orthopedic doctor.

Sophia had diabetes with the side effect of *neuropathy*. Her primary care physician had written a prescription for her shoes, which I was obliged to follow.

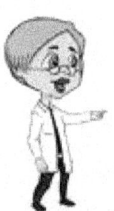
Under the Medicare Diabetic bill, the patient is allowed a shoe style qualified by Medicare and prescribed by a doctor. Diabetic-approved orthotics (a type of supportive, protective arch support with a closed-cell surface) are normally included.

The doctor must write and date the patient's qualifying health conditions in his files as well as on the forms sent in to Medicare.

Usually, if not always, this does not include narrow, pointed shoes!

Sophia arrived with her grown son, his wife, and two grandchildren in tow. They were to be translators for her, but they were there primarily to persuade me to talk her into wearing the shoes the doctor had prescribed for her.

The family had talked until they were exasperated; still she would not give in. The grandchildren had been instructed to plead with her; there had been a few strong conversations with the grown children; and still she held out with arms folded and a mischievous glint in her eye.

So, the family asked me to persuade her to wear the larger toe box shoes. I had met my match with this very clever woman and she was not having any of it.

Sophia was willing to try on any shoe I brought to her, but without giving an explanation, she vetoed each one in turn.

The best I could do was to stretch her shoes on the stretching machine to give her toes more room. I thought they would pop open at the seams. Then I called her physician.

I told the family, including Sophia, that I would be calling her physician for further instruction. Sophia was calm and still smiling, but I thought her son was going to pull his hair out.

Calling Sophia's doctor and recording the situation in Sophia's file, I waited for further instruction.

Several days later, a shoe vendor brought some samples to the store. I immediately thought of Sophia.

These shoes were slim and looked very much like the shoes she was previously wearing, but they had a stretch material built into the leather, disguised by a textured pattern that looked like leather. They were sleek, pretty, and would stretch—relieving pressure and letting air through the important toe box area.

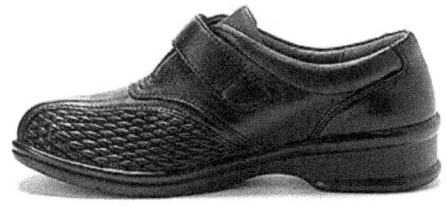

Sophia's new shoe with stretch panels

I immediately called Sophia's doctor for approval. He faxed a new prescription to me and I crossed my fingers that they would pass Sophia's scrutiny.

As soon as the shoes were delivered, I called Sophia's son and invited them back to the store. They arrived within the hour. As I opened the shoe box and took the new shoes out, Sophia looked confused. These shoes were obviously narrower than anything else I had showed her previously. I asked Sophia to stand in the shoes and walk to the floor-length mirror. She turned from side to side, admiring her silhouette, then nodded and told her family they felt good. I got a hug and a wink from Sophia.

The shoes came in other colors, and we agreed she would wear the black shoes for a few weeks and decide if she would like more pairs.

The family returned the following month and Sophia had decided on two more pairs. When I asked her which colors she would like, she told her son, "black." No one tried to talk her into anything else.

Sophia was compliant, safe, and a very stylish woman. **_Salute!_**

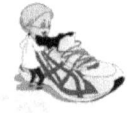

101 Foot Pain

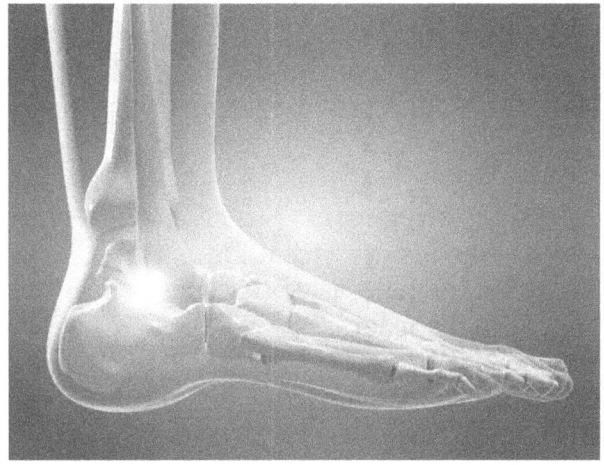

Solutions on a Budget

I Foot Care Basics

When do you need a specialist?

Podiatrists or 'foot doctors', are medical professionals devoted to the study and medical treatment of disorders of the foot, ankle and lower extremity.

Primary care doctors are physicians who provide both the first contact for a person with an undiagnosed health concern as well as continuing care of varied medical conditions, not limited by cause, organ system, or diagnosis

Orthopedic surgeons use both surgical and nonsurgical means to treat musculoskeletal trauma, sports injuries, degenerative diseases, infections, tumors, and congenital disorders.

Dermatologists specialize in the physiology and pathology of the skin.

A **Certified Pedorthist** designs, manufactures, and modifies for fit of footwear, including shoes, orthotics and foot devices, to prevent or alleviate foot problems caused by disease, congenital defect, overuse, or injury.

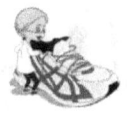

Most footwear prescriptions are written by doctors. In some states, **physical therapists, physicians' assistants, chiropractors, certified pedorthists,** and additional professionals are authorized to write footwear prescriptions.

Problems with feet can be the first sign of more serious medical conditions such as:

Arthritis, joint, and bone disease
Diabetes or high blood pressure
Nerve disease due to neuropathy
Circulatory disorders such as ulcers, cellulitis, neuritis, vascular insufficiency, and gangrene

Years of sports and weight gain age your feet, as well as disease, poor circulation, improperly trimmed toenails, and wearing shoes that don't fit properly.

Practice good foot care. Check your feet regularly, or have a member of your family check them. A mirror under your feet with a good, bright light can allow you to check the bottoms of your feet.

Keep the blood circulating in your feet as much as possible. Do this by putting your feet up when you are sitting or lying down, stretching if you have to sit for a long while, walking, having a gentle foot massage (yes, you can do it yourself) or taking a warm foot bath.

Avoid pressure from shoes that don't fit right.
Try not to expose your feet to cold temperatures.
Don't sit for long periods of time (especially with your legs crossed).
Don't smoke.

Dirty Feet: It is easy to get cracked heels from the heat of the summer months and the dry air in the winter. Dirt and grime can get into those cracks and make feet look dirty.

After washing your feet with a good, moisturizing soap, soak your feet in water with an equal part Listerine and water for about 30 minutes.

Rub with a net sponge or a rough towel.

Apply foot cream or lotion regularly. Moisturize the rough spots on your feet every night.

Make sure your feet are good and dry before putting on your socks and shoes.

Washing your feet in the shower: This can be a *real pain* when you can't bend over, don't have the strength to stand and support yourself, or don't have the balance needed to accomplish this without falling on your head.

Many people would love to wash their feet sitting in the bathtub, but alas, the same problems surface. They can't be secure enough in their strength and balance to step over the side of the tub or to lift themselves up from the tub bottom or the side of the tub.

So, if you need to get your feet clean, avoid fungus infections, clean grime away so you don't start growing a garden between your toes, or want to feel proud when someone looks at your pedicure, you could try this idea:

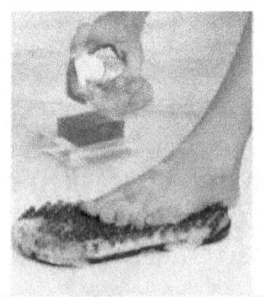

Bathtub foot scrubber

Go to a medical supply store that sells canes, crutches, stocking-donners, etc. Generally they will have a flat plastic surface that has suction cups on the bottom and a short, plastic brush surface on top.

The brush surface should be firm, but soft. You will be able to stand, holding onto the wall or a safety bar, and pour some liquid body wash onto the brush surface.

Wet your feet under the shower stream and brush your feet back and forth, side to side, to wash the sides and bottoms of your feet. Rinse and admire those pretty little piggies!

I have seen these devices at Walgreen, Walmart, and even the Dollar Store on occasion. Keep your eyes open.

Drying between your toes is important, especially if you are diabetic. If you don't have any help, you can sit down, hold each end of a towel, and slide your feet around on it while it is on the floor.

Another good plan is to use your blow dryer set on warm, not hot, to blow the moisture away. Make sure your feet are good and dry, especially between your toes, before applying lotions and putting on your socks and shoes.

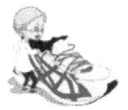

Homemade Foot Soak Recipes

Water temperature is a personal preference. Do not use hot water if you have neuropathy. People with diabetes should not soak their feet.

Directions: thoroughly mix all of the following ingredients, then store in an airtight container. Use 2 to 3 tablespoons per gallon of water.

Basic Recipe
1 part Epsom salts
1 part baking soda
Several drops of quality scented body oils

Tea bags, milk, olive oil, and honey can be added for varying effects.

Adding marbles or round stones to the soak can provide a soothing massage as you gently roll your feet against them.

If you are diabetic and/or have neuropathy, consult your doctor before trying new foot treatments. Examine your feet frequently.

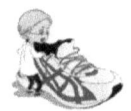

Sweaty, smelly feet: Foot odor, known in the medical profession as bromhidrosis, is caused by bacteria that find your moist, warm socks and shoes a perfect place to breed.

The foot has many sweat glands and these glands produce fats, minerals, and secretions that can produce a foul odor.

Wash your feet well with deodorant soap and completely dry them. Some people with the worst odors wash their feet several times a day. Watch for scaly and cracked skin, as there must be naturally-occurring protective oil on the skin. This means cutting back on the number of washings.

Sea salt in warm water may be a good remedy. If you soak the foot in this mixture and let them dry without rinsing, the feet will stay dry for longer.

Bacteria-killing deodorant or antiperspirant can be used on the feet as well as the armpits. The deodorant won't dry them up, but killing the bacteria will kill the odor and the antiperspirant will help keep the feet dry.

Change your socks: Do not wear the same pair of socks for two days in a row. If you are diabetic with neuropathy, you should change your socks throughout the day, both to inspect your feet and to change the places on your foot where a sock may bunch and create a fold or a seam that could be causing pressure.

Leather shoes or open weave shoes will breathe and help keep feet dry. Some open weave fabrics or canvas shoes can be washed in the washing machine.

Exchange your shoes with another pair in your closet. Let the first ones dry out and decompress. They will smell better and last longer. If you can set them out on a porch or deck, the sunshine and fresh air will help kill the bacteria hiding inside.

Powders and cornstarch can help keep things dry. Foot powders can be put on the feet and cornstarch sprinkled in the shoes.

Even stress and the foods you eat can come through the sweat glands and change your body odor. Try to calm down and avoid strong foods such as onion, garlic, bleu cheese, etc....

Dry skin and cracked heels can cause itching and burning feet. Use mild soap in small amounts, and a moisturizing cream or lotion on your legs and feet every day.

Alcohol-based products can dry out your skin. Be careful about adding oils to bathwater, because they can make your feet and bathtub very slippery.

Another solution is oil-releasing slippers/socks for soft, moisturized feet. Many shoe stores, along with variety and department stores, sell slippers that are lined inside with different oils embedded in a light gel lining. The slippers/socks are worn at night during sleep. Wake up with soft, smooth skin.

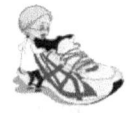

II Shoe Fit and Maintenance

Tips for getting a proper shoe fit:

Wear comfortable shoes that fit well. The size of your feet changes as you grow older, so always have your feet measured before buying shoes. The best time to measure your feet is at the end of the day, when your feet are largest.

Fit your shoe to your larger foot. Most of us have one foot larger than the other. Don't select shoes by the size marked inside the shoe but by how the shoe fits your foot.

Select a shoe that is shaped like your foot. Have someone draw an outline of your feet while you stand on a piece of paper. Take the cut out outlines with you to the shoe store help you at the shoe store. Turn the shoes of your choice upside down and apply your outlines to the bottoms. Do the shoes look too narrow or short beneath the cutouts?

Make sure there is enough space (3/8" to 1/2"), or a thumb width, for your longest toe at the end of each shoe when you are standing up. Your foot will push forward as you take each step.

Make sure the ball of your foot fits comfortably in the widest part of the shoe. Don't buy shoes that feel too tight and expect them to stretch to fit.

Your heel should fit comfortably in the shoe with a minimum amount of slipping. The shoes should not ride up and down on your heel when you walk unless they are built like a Dansko clog, which is intended to slip.

Walk in the shoes to make sure they fit and feel right; then take them home and spend some time walking on carpet to make sure the fit is a good one. Most shoe stores will allow you to bring them back if the shoes look new and can be resold; ask about their policy.

Choose proper shoe materials. The upper part of the shoes should be made of a soft, flexible material to match the shape of your foot. Shoes made of leather can reduce the possibility of skin irritations.

Soles should provide solid footing and not be slippery. Thick soles will cushion your feet when you walk on hard surfaces. Low-heeled shoes are more comfortable, safer, and less damaging than high-heeled shoes.

Squeaks can be caused, primarily, by a custom-made, plastic orthotic, or a hard cork arch support. Squeaking sounds are caused when two dissimilar materials rub together.

Let's say you buy a pair of sandals that have a soft cushion arch support and you need to replace the soft arch supports with the cork-bed that you took from another pair of shoes. The interior of the sandals where the original arch support fit is black rubber inside leather sandals.

The cork arch supports were inside a solid leather interior. Now the cork arch support squeaks with each step against the black rubber sandal interior. What do you do?

One good solution is to use *sandpaper* or a small grinding tool with sander disks to gently rough up the edges of the cork bed. Don't take too much off, just rough up the surface. This will create friction that will keep the arch support in place.

Another possibility is to use *baby powder* to coat the inside of the sandal bed. This will act as a lubricant to let the two surfaces slide against each other.

Don't give up; you can fix a squeaker!

Shrinking stretched leather: When a favorite, well-worn pair of shoes has gotten too loose, stretching them can save your money and comfort.

A shoe is made from wet leather, stretched around a shoe form (called a "last") and then dried with hot air. As the damp leather dries, it takes the shape of the shoe-form, tightening and smoothing the leather.

When you have a stretched, loose shoe, the shoe can be put back on a shoe stretcher or stuffed firmly with cloth or paper and sprayed with an alcohol-based shoe-stretch fluid.

A hot blow dryer can be used to heat the leather. Take care not to burn the shoe or the hands holding the shoe. As the leather heats, it will start tightening. Let the shoe cool down before handling or putting on the foot.

Breaking in new shoes by hand can shorten the time it takes to be comfortable and can save you from blisters. A common problem with new shoes is that the heel and sole are too stiff to bend correctly at the ball of the foot. This makes the heel pull and sometimes slip up and down.

The form, or "cup," inside the back of the heel is made of plastic. Wearing a pair of gloves, you can heat the heel cup inside the shoe with a hot blow dryer.

The cup will be more pliable. Immediately you can push the top, back of the heel and bend it back and forth to make the heel much more flexible and comfortable.

Without the heat, you can firmly hold the toe of the shoe in one hand and the heel in the other and bend the shoe in half where the ball of the foot would be. Flexing the shoe back and forth in this area will make walking so much more comfortable and help keep the heel where it should be.

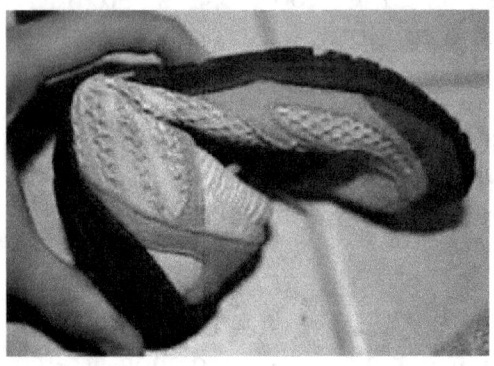

Bending a new shoe sole to be more flexible

Flip-flops

> "With a litany of stubbed toes, sprained ankles, broken bones and blistered feet, Americans' feet are hurting. According to the National Foot Health Assessment 2012 released in June, 2013, "78% of adults 21 and older have experienced one or more foot problems in their lives."
>
> —CNN

No heel support, no structural support, no arch support; just a little piece of rubber.

Concrete, asphalt, and steel cover our world today. These are hard surfaces to walk on barefoot. There isn't anything to absorb the impact and shock when you walk in a pair of flip-flops.

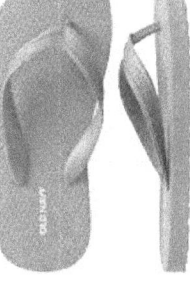

Flip-flops

Although feet were designed to walk barefoot on Earth's natural surfaces (grass, sand, or dirt), they were not prepared to endure the concrete, asphalt, and steel that covers so many landscapes today. These hard surfaces are harsh on bare feet, and the thin rubber soles of many flip-flops do little to absorb the shock they produce.

Whether you are standing still or in motion, your feet are your first point of contact with the ground.

The positioning of your feet determines the body's skeletal alignment. Flip-flops have little arch support and over time could lead to pain in the knees, hips, and back.

Flip-flops can lead to falls, twisted ankles, and broken bones.

> ***People with diabetes should never wear plain flip-flops. Feet can get cuts, scrapes, and bruises which may not heal quickly, if at all.***

Look for a pair with deep heel cups, high arch support, and comfortable toe support if you are in a condition to wear open-toe shoes. There are many brands out there that will help with support.

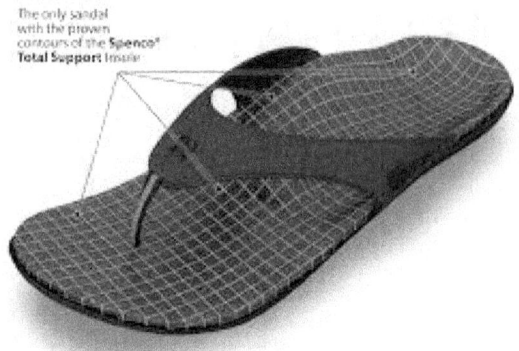

Spenco flip-flops with arch support and deep heel cup

As people have gained weight over the years, it is even more important to have support for the extra strain put on the joints and tendons.

Flip-flops can be beneficial in guarding against bacterial and fungal infections at gyms and pools as well as protecting the foot from hot sand at the beach.

Crocs could be a better alternative to give the foot some protection if the lighter-weight shoe feels like a necessity.

Be sure to wash your feet well after taking them off, and inspect your feet frequently.

Mismatched shoes: Everyone's feet are mismatched to a degree. That is normal, but when the size difference becomes too great, the smaller foot will slip and slide inside the shoe unless it's filled with a lot of material.

Often the arch will not be in the right spot and sometimes the size difference is in the width or girth of the foot and not the length.

It can get expensive to buy two pairs of shoes in different sizes, but that is an option if the company doesn't sell mismatched shoes. There are places to donate new mismatched shoes for people with amputations.
To learn more visit:

www.waterfrontmission.org/recycling-donation-centers

If your nonprofit or charitable organization would like to learn more about the benefits of establishing a recycling program, send an email to:
admin@waterfrontmission.org

Type "RECYCLING INFORMATION REQUEST" in the subject line of your email.

Ask your shoe clerk if they have a shoe vendor who will sell mismatched shoes. Most of the time, you will pay one and one-half times the cost of a normal pair of shoes instead of the full price for two pair.

Old Friend Step-in Slippers open up completely with Velcro fasteners. This is a great help to people suffering from lymphedema (fluid buildup and heavy swelling) in the lower extremities or if a thick bandage must be worn around the foot. This slipper has leather outer with sheep fleece lining inside. They are very comfortable for most people.

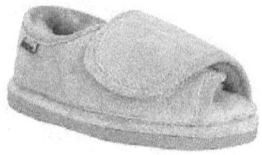

Old Friend Step-in Slippers

If all else fails, polish them! Have you ever had a pair of suede or Nubuck shoes that had something spilled on them or spots from walking through snow? Maybe the sun has bleached one more than the other.

If no cleaner will get it out, you can polish them. No, they will not have the "nappy" feel or appearance anymore, but the polish will soak in and then coat the shoe to even out the colors. You will then be able to buff them with a shoe brush. Don't throw away a good pair of shoes that look bad; try this trick instead.

Water-wicking socks pull the perspiration away from the skin and let the moisture evaporate so the feet won't dry and crack, or host bacteria and fungi.

Dark, warm, wet places are favorite breeding grounds of bacteria and fungi, especially between the toes. This is another good reason to wear shoes with adequate toe box room so that the skin can "breathe" and have air circulation.

Water-wicking socks can be found in most shoe stores now, as well as in sports and camping stores.

D-I-Y arch supports can be made from a variety of materials.

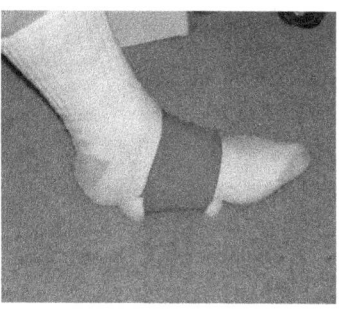

Homemade arch supports

These creative slip-on arch supports are made from a grout sponge and red stretch material, using a tube sized for the diameter of their foot to measure the red stretch band. They sewed a pocket for the sponge to keep it in place.

This kind of support usually works better turned under the arch more and brought back toward the heel.

This solution will not take the place of a doctor's recommendation.

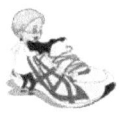

III Solutions for Foot Health Problems

Achilles tendonitis is very painful and can make it hard to find any shoes that are comfortable. The Achilles tendon runs down the back of the heel. A tight tendon can also contribute to plantar fasciitis, another painful condition on the bottom (plantar) side of the foot.

Several things can be done to relieve the pressure on the inflamed tendon. A soft pad can be applied inside the back heel of the shoe. A horseshoe shaped pad can allow the tendon to be offloaded from the pressure of the plastic cup inside the heel.

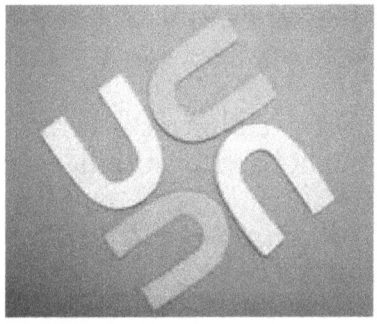

Pads cut like horse shoes

If none of the pads for Achilles tendonitis relieve pain and pressure, the plastic heel cup might need to be removed. The cup is sandwiched between the inner and outer layers of the back of the heel area. After the cup is removed, the layers can be glued or sewn back together. A shoe repair shop can easily do this for you.

Arthritis and degenerative joint disease refers to wear and tear on a joint. This condition is usually brought on by injury, but can also be caused by metabolic abnormalities, infections, tumors, or deformities.

The condition continues to get worse. X-rays can determine the severity of disease. Sometimes the symptoms don't seem to match the results of the x-rays, though.

Motion control or immobilizing the joint, ibuprofen, or other anti-inflammatories, rest, compression, and elevation can help at the onset of the condition.

If surgery is needed, there may be cleaning of the joint "bone debris," joint replacement, or fusion of the joint to modify painful movement.

Athlete's foot is a fungal infection that can cause peeling, redness, itching, burning, and sometimes blisters and sores. Athlete's foot is mildly contagious, passed by direct contact or by walking barefoot in areas such as locker rooms, or near pools. Our feet spend a lot of time in shoes - a warm, dark, humid place that is perfect for fungus to grow, especially if the shoes are made of a man-made material.

To prevent infections, keep your feet, especially between your toes, clean and dry. Change your shoes and socks or stockings often to help keep your feet dry. You can use foot powder daily, but, if your foot condition does not get better in two weeks, talk to your doctor.

Bunion or hallux valgus is a condition of the big toe. The joint at the base of the toe looks like it has a bump growing on the side of this joint (metatarsophalangeal or MTP joint).

The big toe begins to point toward the outside of the foot and the toe bone just above the first joint begins to angle in toward the rest of the toes.

First a callus can form and then the bone can thicken as a response to pressure and rubbing against the swollen tissue caught between the inside of the shoe and the deformed joint. The bunion forms from the pressure from the shoe at the deformed big toe joint.

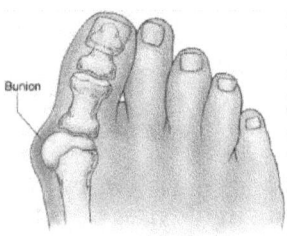

Bunion

This toe deformity becomes a cosmetic and fashion problem. Even when wearing sandals, the bunion can protrude between the straps of leather—looking unsightly.

Slender-toed shoes can be unbearable due to the pressure of the shoe against the bunion. High-heeled shoes cause the forefoot to bear weight and put more stress on the deformed joint forming the bunion. As the problem worsens, the second toe can move upward, and may constantly be rubbing on the top of the shoe. Cultures that go barefoot don't normally get bunions.

Wide shoes with plenty of room for the toes, unlike high heels and pointed boots, help reduce the irritation.

Pain relievers: There are several types of bunion pads to cushion the bunion: toe spacers, toe splints, and custom shoe inserts.

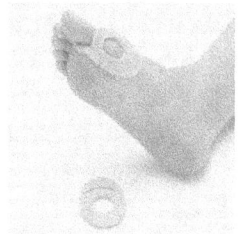

Slip-on toe bunion cut outs

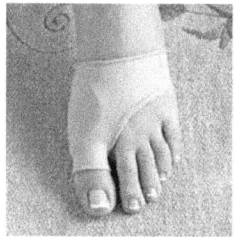

Slip-on bunion pad

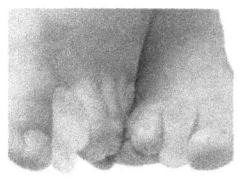

Gel toe spacers

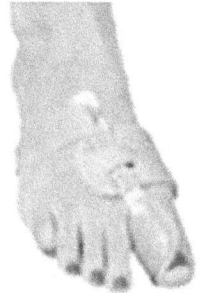

Night time bunion splint

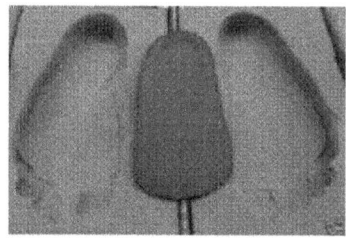

Custom-made orthotics

Surgery may help the condition. X-rays would be ordered by your doctor as he or she measures the angle of the toe joint's deformity for a conclusive course of action.

There are well over 100 surgical procedures to treat hallux valgus (condition causing bunions). In some very mild cases of bunion formation, surgery may only be required to remove the bunion itself.

The major decision that must be made is whether or not the metatarsal bone will need to be cut and re-aligned as well. The bone is re-aligned and held in place with metal pins until it heals as well as balance the conditions so the bunion does not return. It will take about eight weeks before the bones and soft tissues are healed after surgery.

The top of your foot is called the "instep." Some people have particularly bony feet. Not much "padding" on these people. Sometimes their arches are higher than average, a condition called a pes cavus arch; a "cave" forms under the arch!

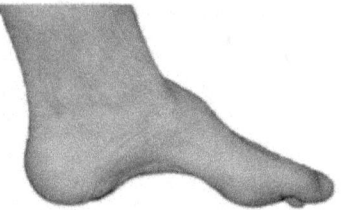

Pes cavus Arch

For this type of foot, shoe strings can be a curse. The overzealous store clerk may tie them too tight, bruising and irritating the tendons and bones above the instep.

An extra pad may be attached under the tongue of the shoe before tying the shoes. It is best to choose tie shoes that have a tongue, so a pad can be attached that will sit against the boney instep.

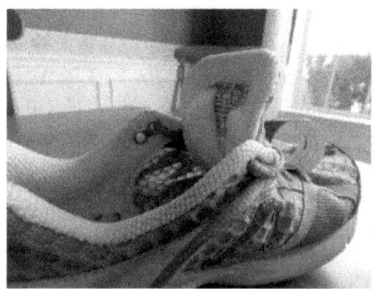

Extra padding attached under tongue of shoe

Where can you get that pad? Be creative. Many orthopedic shoe stores have flat, dense cotton pads with a sticky back to attach to the shoe.

Craft stores have flat dense foam in 8-by-10-inch sheets. The sheets can be cut to just the right size and glued in place or attached with double-stick tape.

Panty liners, felt squares, or new shoe liners can all be cut to shape and size as needed.

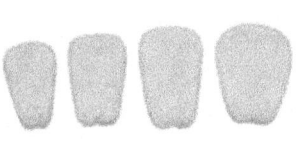

Pre-made pads

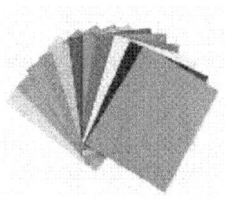

Foam Art store pads

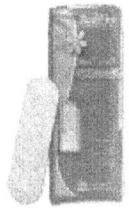

Panty liners

When wearing something new in your shoe, treat it like wearing a new shoe. Break in slowly and continue checking the area of contact to make sure you are not getting a blister.

As usual, use good sense and contact your health care provider with any questions or concerns.

Steel and plastic toe protectors both have their purpose. For many years, steel-toe boots have been the only choice for people working in construction or industrial areas. Many companies require them in order to get the job.
People with diabetes are usually discouraged from wearing steel toe boots or shoes. Many companies now make plastic composite toe boxes that have a comparable durability to steel toes.

The best feature of these newer plastic composite toes is that they can be made higher and wider to give the foot more room with less chance of toes rubbing against the toe protector and creating an injury just from wearing the shoes.

Ask your favorite shoe store about this possibility. Don't forget, if necessary, several companies will make modified shoes, including special chemical resistant soles.

Flatfoot (pes planus) occurs when the sole of the foot comes into near-complete contact with the ground. Inherited, caused by injury, or a condition such as rheumatoid arthritis, treatment includes foot-strengthening exercises, and shoes with good arch support or orthotics. Flatfoot condition rarely causes problems, but sometimes badly fitting shoes, weight-gain, or sudden athletic activity may cause pain.

Gout is a form of arthritis. Sudden pain, redness, swelling, and stiffness, usually in the large joint of the big toe, can alert your physician to an onset of gout. Gout can also occur in other joints of the body. Too much uric acid (UA) in the body can form hard crystals in joints. Gout attacks can last days or weeks, and may be treated with anti-inflammatories or medication to lower uric acid. The physician may change a patient's diet to help break down UA.

Hammertoes and claw toes are similar, because a person with this condition ultimately ends up pushing off on the tips of their toes. Those tender areas were not built to take the pressure. Often one of the toes ends up crossing over another one or two toes, causing more pain and problems walking.

When toe muscles get out of balance, they can cause painful toe problems. While some people are prone to hammertoe, other risks include tight footwear. Hammertoe generally causes the middle joint of the toe to bend downward, with toes appearing raised near the foot. Well-fitted footwear with the correct amount of space in the toe box, shoe supports, and surgery may offer relief.

Terms and medical descriptions involve hyper flexion deformity of the proximal interphalangeal (PIP) joint, hyper flexion, PIP joint, and the metatarsal phalangeal (MTP) joint. Most of you are not inclined to have medical degrees, so here are a couple of pictures of the condition.

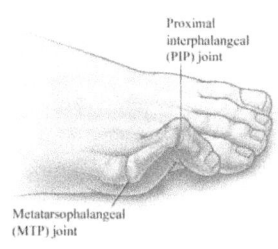

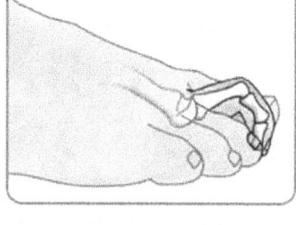

Hammer Toes

Claw Toes

Hammer Toes are a fairly common condition in cultures that wear shoes. In most cases, the problem can be traced to improper shoes!

Hammertoes are likely the result of a shoe that is too pointed or too short. Combine pointed shoes with high heels and the toes are pushed into a deformed position. Day after day the tendons of the toes shorten and tighten due to the contraction of the toes. The toes become fixed in that position, resembling a claw, and will not straighten out. Pressure builds up at the toe joints (PIP and MTP) and at the end of the toe, causing calluses and blisters, and sometimes ulcers, to develop.

Testing can show that no other problems of the nerves are causing this condition and treatment depends on how severely the problem has developed.

If the joints of the toe are still flexible, changing to a better fitting shoe can allow the toes to relax and return close to normal again. If the toes are already rigid, shoes with a higher and wider toe box plus soft padding will keep the tops of the hammer toes from getting sores.

The padded devices shown below reduce pressure on the tips of the toes or protect the top of the raised toes. Be careful and don't pull the elastic band too tight! You don't want to cut off the blood circulation to the toe.

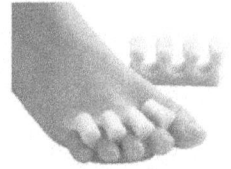
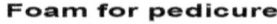

Foam for pedicure

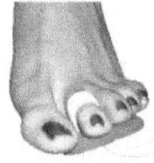

Hammer toe pads

If all else fails, surgery may be suggested to correct the alignment of the toe. Checking with several facilities before your surgery can be smart. There can be a significant difference in the charges. Unexpected things may alter the estimated price, but a good estimate can at least give you an idea and a basis for comparison.

Ingrown toenails can feel like a toothache in your toe! Ouch! Redness, feverish swelling, and pain are the symptoms. Wearing shoes that are too tight can exacerbate the situation.

As it is a very painful and common ailment, many home remedies have been used and handed down over the years. Very few will work, as they normally involve self-surgery of sorts.

One procedure that has some promise of note is to lift the ingrown toenail corner away from the toe and stuff a small piece of cotton under the edge of the offending toenail and nail channel. The idea is for the nail to grow up and over the cotton until it gets beyond the end of the toe bed.

Several surgical procedures for ingrown toenails have been developed by medical professionals over time.

An older method was to remove the offending part of the nail and scrape the nail growing plate completely down to the bone. This method incapacitates the patient for a week to 10 days and there is more risk of infection.

There was a time when laser surgery was thought to be the best answer, but the laser is used to burn the nail-growth cells. The trauma to the area and the recovery time are much more than expected. The laser also neglects to destroy all the nail-growth cells, so the offending ingrown toenail can grow back over time.

The final procedure is a surgery that does not require the toe to be "opened." This is the *phenol-and-alcohol* method. A mixture is used to kill the plate-growth-cells and a disinfectant is applied to prevent bacterial infection in the area of the surgery. The procedure only takes a few minutes.

The patient can walk with surgical sandals immediately after the procedure. The risk of infection is low and people who are diabetic and have circulatory issues may do very well with this procedure. *Ask your health care provider for your best options.*

Leg length discrepancy means one leg is longer than the other. Usually the shorter leg will start feeling the effects first: anything from patella (knee cap) pain to pelvis pain and many more side effects.

There are a few ways to measure for LLD. The physician can examine a person or take an x-ray.

Using wooden blocks of different height, the patient can stand on each of the thicknesses under the shorter leg.

Continuing to measure the belt line, the examiner can tell how thick the leg lift should be.

Another way to measure is from the iliac crest (top of the hip bone) to the floor and the bump on the outside of the ankle (fibula) to the floor on each leg. This will take into account a flat foot with a fallen arch on one side.

The picture below shows a device that can be strapped to the patient's own shoe. Different thicknesses of dense material are added under the shoe so the patient can walk around with the different height lifts while they are again measured.

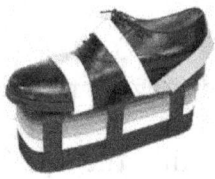

Leg length discrepancy tester

Depending on how much lift is needed, a simple heel lift can be inserted into the shoe under the heel. If half an inch or more is needed, the lift should be added to the bottom of the shoe. If more than this thickness is added under the heel, it will make the patient walk in a "high-heeled" position, putting too much pressure and stress on the front of the foot and causing the back to be out of alignment.

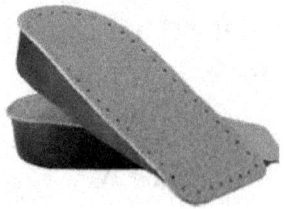

Adjustable thickness heel lifts

Morton's neuroma is a nerve inflammation between the third and fourth toes. Do you have burning, tingling, aching pain radiating into two adjacent toes? You may have a neuroma.

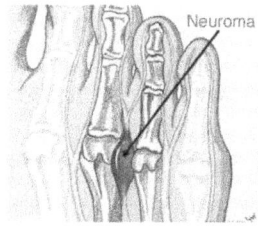

Morton's neuroma inflamed nerve

A nerve between two toes in the forefoot becomes inflamed. This could be caused by wearing shoes that are too tight, high heels, or an injury to the foot. The inflamed, swollen area is caused by abnormal growth of nerve cells from the irritation of the nerve.

Sometimes the doctor will do a test called the *Mulder's sign* to make sure it is a neuroma and not another problem. This test is no fun.

Already experiencing a sharp, knife-like feeling in the bottom of the foot and generalized aching and pain, the doctor will squeeze the forefoot, listening for a "popping" sound and probably your loud cursing. The louder the pop sounds, the larger the neuroma.

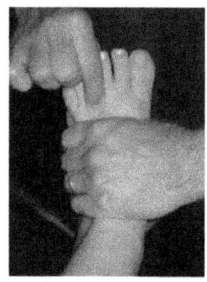

Mulder's sign

There are many different treatment options according to the severity of the neuroma and the pain it is causing.

Your doctor may decide to try a cortisone injection with an anesthetic into the area of the inflamed nerve.

Change shoes. Are your shoes too tight? Are they high heels? Do they force you to walk in an odd way with pressure on your forefoot and no padding and support? If they cause your feet to hurt this much...give them or throw them away, *permanently*.

A variety of pads in soft, compressed wool, silicone gel, or a firm sponge material could be used for a metatarsal pad. They are cut to lift behind the affected area and to relieve the pressure on the neuroma. You can try cutting a thick spongy shoe insert into these shapes.

Some orthopedic or retail shoe stores will sell these outright for you to install yourself, or you may negotiate with one of their pedorthists to do it for you. A thin Kotex pad can be cut to shape and tacked in the shoe with double-stick tape.

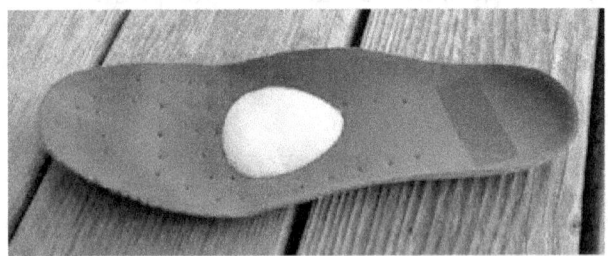

Morton's neuroma pad

A serious option for Morton's neuroma is surgery, but **nerve surgery** can be tricky and not always productive. Again,

110

your health provider will help you make the best decisions for your condition.

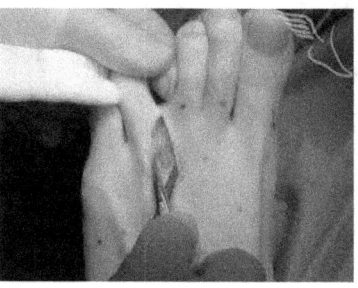

Morton's neuroma surgery

Morton's toe occurs when your second or third toe is longer than your big toe. Really push those toes flat to compare. Are you wearing shoes to accommodate the LONGEST toe or toes?

Feet shift forward a bit when you take a step. You need a little room for that. Many people are walking around with a size 8 shoe on a size 9 foot. Be your own shoe clerk and get some relief!

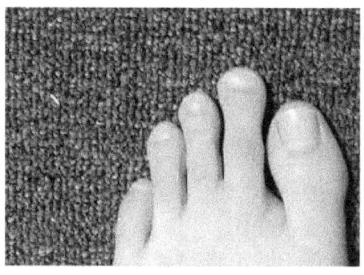

Morton's Toe

Over pronation is the reason for 98% of biomechanical foot problems. Only about 2% are caused by over-supination. Most true supination problems are caused by neuromuscular disorders requiring a specialist to treat them.

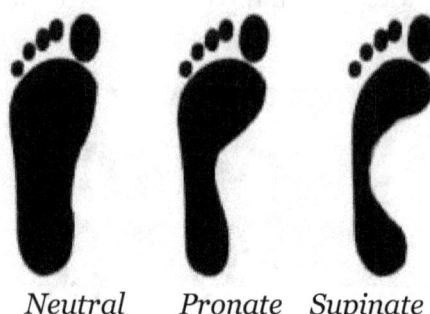

Neutral   Pronate   Supinate

Normal feet do both pronation and supination as a person takes a step (the gait cycle). It is **abnormal** pronation or supination that causes the problems.

Plantar fasciitis/heel spurs symptoms usually occur when you step from bed in the middle of the night, and in the morning, but can occur after sitting down for a few minutes or more.

Usually symptoms improve as the arch and calf muscle stretch to a normal position. This is why stretching is an important part of the treatment plan. Your body weight, foot type, shoe-design and occupation may all be contributing causes of this condition. Diagnosis can be made during the physical examination. X-rays could be taken to rule out an underlying cause such as other injury or inflammatory disease.

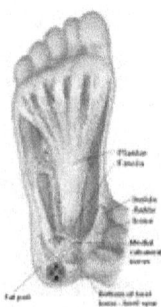

Sharp pain with first step out of bed

112

The red spot with "X" notes attachment of plantar fascia to the heel bone. This is a common area for sharp pain upon rising for the first step in the morning when you have Plantar fasciitis.

X-rays may show a heel spur i.e., Heel Spur Syndrome but, the spur has never been proven to be the actual cause of pain.

Spurs are calcium growths that develop on the bones of your feet. They are caused by muscle strain in the feet. Standing a lot, wearing shoes that don't fit, or gaining too much weight can make spurs worse. Spurs can be completely painless or very painful. Helpful treatments for bone spurs include arch supports, heel-pads, and heel cups, or surgery if necessary.

Treatment for plantar fasciitis includes injection, taping, orthotics, physical therapy, anti-inflammatory medications and ice, night-splinting, and surgical techniques including endoscopic plantar fasciotomy.

A newer treatment utilizes sound waves to create new blood vessels at the painful area, and has been shown to be very effective. Energy sound waves are showing promise. The higher the energy wave, the more effective the treatment can be. It is a good alternative to surgery.

Plantar warts are tough growths that grow on the soles of the feet. They are caused by a virus entering through broken skin, and are often spread through public pools and showers.

Plantar warts are harmless, but sometimes they are too painful to ignore. Topical salicylic acid may help. Burning, freezing, using laser therapy and surgical removal may be necessary for more severe cases. *Don't use anything until checking with your doctor, especially if you are diabetic!*

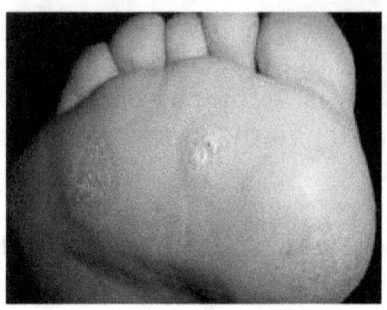

Plantar wart

Pregnancy

"A natural hormone, **elastin**, is released during pregnancy. This hormone works to gradually relax the ligaments connecting the pubic bones, which helps to accommodate for delivery.

Elastin also affects another important ligament (the Spring ligament) located in your feet, causing it to relax and stretch. This results in less support for the arch and a gradual flattening of the feet. This condition is aggravated by weight gain during pregnancy. As your arch provides less and less support, you experience increased strain on your feet, knees and the muscles in your lower back. Ultimately, this can cause discomfort in the joints of your feet and lower back muscles."

—Dr. Ivar Roth, Podiatrist and Foot & Ankle Surgeon

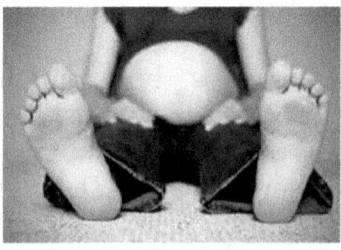

Pregnant women's foot size increases
114

Have you ever overheard a woman say, "I don't know what happened, I gained two shoe sizes since my pregnancy!" Elastin is one of the reasons. The foot should be supported so the arches don't gradually flatten, leaving you with a larger size foot!

> *"We are taking the 'visit to the doctor' out of the equation to help more people solve their own foot problems."*
>
> —Dr. Ivar Roth, Podiatrist and Foot & Ankle Surgeon

Dr. Roth recommends a product that he sells on the internet called "FABS." They are a wrap-around device with Velcro and an attached pad to be worn for arch support. This can also help with plantar fasciitis.

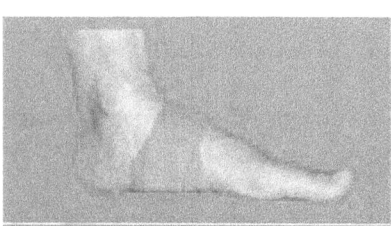 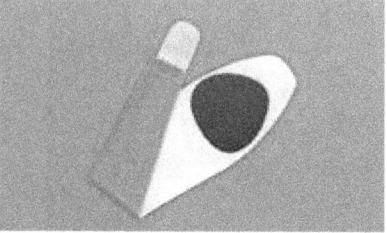

FABS

Tendonitis is a common problem of the foot. The *posterior tibial tendon* most often causes tendonitis. Behind the inside bump on the ankle (*medial malleolus*) it runs across the instep to the bottom of the foot (the *plantar* side). This tendon helps to support the arch of the foot and to turn the foot inward to keep the foot straight when we walk.

As we age and continue daily walking, there is some degeneration (wear and tear) of the tendon. This leads to the tendon being weaker than it should be.

When a person has tendonitis of the posterior tibial tendon, a painful instep will result with swelling along the path of the tendon. The tendon may rupture, due to weakening of the tendon from inflammation. If the tendon ruptures, it will let the arches collapse and cause a significant and recognizable flat foot.

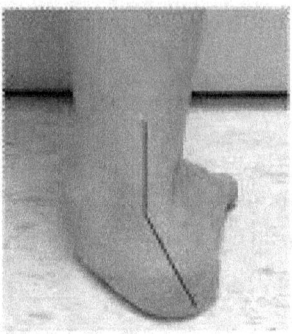

Posterial tibial tendon has ruptured

(Picture is from the back of the heel. The line is to show angle).

Treatment of this condition before getting to the rupture stage begins with a good arch support. This takes some of the stress off the tendon. Decreasing activity may be necessary, to rest the tendon. Anti-inflammatory medications, such as ibuprofen or aspirin, may be prescribed by your physician.

If the tendon has ruptured, surgery may be required to either repair the ruptured tendon, or in cases that have gone untreated, the bones in the foot may have to be fused together.

Following surgery, the patient's foot may be placed in a brace or cast. The patient will have to probably be in a cast for 6-8 weeks if a fusion has been performed.

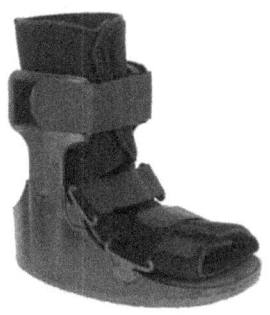

Surgical walking boot

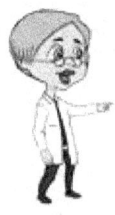

***Please consult your physician if you
are experiencing pain in these areas***

Toenail fungus gets started when microscopic fungi enter through a break or tear in the nail. It can make your nails thick, brittle, and dark colored. This fungus likes warm, wet places and other people can get it from you.

Getting rid of toenail fungus can be a challenge. If caught early enough, topical creams may take care of it.

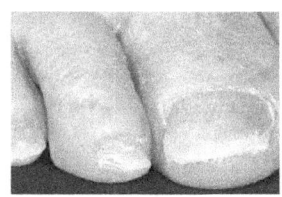

Toenail fungus

Many people with toenail fungus walk around smelling like eucalyptus oil from Vicks VapoRub, tea tree oil, oregano spirits, or a vinegar solution.

Foot care nurses often hand out this advice. Apply one of the solutions listed above on and around the toe nail to fight the fungus if it has not progressed too far. Any of these should be discontinued if they cause any skin irritation. Some magazines you get in the mail, as well as some local drugstores, will sell fungus ointments.

The next progression of solutions involves a doctor excising the infected nail and then the topical solutions are applied several times per day. The doctor may decide to take only a portion of the nail, depending on how and where the fungus is localized.

Fifty percent of the time, it will take an oral medication to really kill it, and after taking the oral medication for about three months, it can still take 18 months for the fungus to die, working 80% of the time.

Keeping the toes and feet clean and dry in the first place is a good preventative measure as all medicine has side effects.

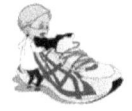

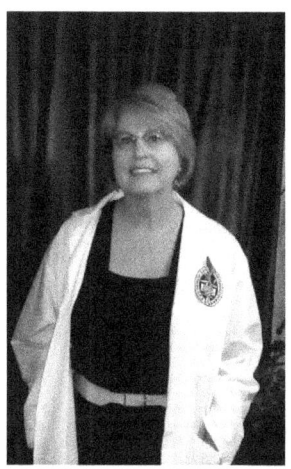

Dear reader,

Thank you for sharing your time with me. As you have seen, foot problems can become big problems. I hope you have found this book helpful and educational, as well as entertaining.

For further questions, feel free to contact me at:

www.footfixes.com
info@footfixes.com

Lynda Elliott Goyzueta
Certified Pedorthist

This book is also available on Amazon Kindle